T0372494

PROZAC
MONOLOGUES

PROZAC MONOLOGUES

A VOICE FROM THE EDGE
WILLA GOODFELLOW

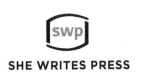

SHE WRITES PRESS

Published 2020
Printed in the United States of America
ISBN: 978-1-63152-731-9
ISBN: 978-1-63152-732-6
Library of Congress Control Number: 2020906458

For information, address:
She Writes Press
1569 Solano Ave #546
Berkeley, CA 94707

Interior design by Tabitha Lahr

She Writes Press is a division of SparkPoint Studio, LLC.

I wrote this for you.

CONTENTS

THE POINT

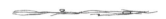

I pressed the point of my nail file into my thumb. Unmindful of the garage attendant as I passed him, unmindful of the cars in the circular drive in front of my doctor's office, unmindful of the ice under my feet, I wondered, could I take a nail file with me on the plane to Costa Rica?

January 4, 2005, the TSA was starting to loosen the rules. Yes, you could carry a nail file, but it would be confiscated if they changed their minds next week. And you'd probably not find out until you were at the airport.

Honestly, could a nail file do any damage? For now, I pressed it into my thumb, intending to do my nails while I waited for the doctor, something to channel my fidgeting. I was fidgeting lately.

The automatic doors slid open to receive me, and my brain slid open to receive a thought.

I grab my doctor from behind and press the point of the nail file into her neck.

This was no ordinary thought. I didn't have this thought. It had me. It was more like a dream and I was inside it. I *saw* it happen inside my head.

Did anybody else see me do that?

Suddenly the reception area was hostile territory. Well, the receptionist was notoriously hostile. But now the doors were too. They'd opened to receive me, but would they release me if they knew about this thought?

Did they know about this thought?

I didn't do my nails. I hid the file. I wouldn't pull it on my doctor anyway. There was a big church meeting coming up in ten days, and I had to be there. I was the priest.

Most clergy wish we didn't have so many meetings to attend. But we usually manage to show up for the ones we are supposed to lead. At this point I was still one of those clergy.

I recited my tale of woe to the doctor. After two months' worth of Prozac to treat a long-term major depression, yes, I was less sad. But now I wasn't sleeping, couldn't concentrate, couldn't work, felt agitated and irritated. I didn't used to feel irritated. I didn't mention the nail file. I wanted those doors to open again and let me out. She figured, and I figured, we needed to increase the dose. Which we did.

A week later I was driving to my congregation, eighty miles south from Iowa City to Fort Madison, through farm fields covered in snow, a rare winter blue sky that day. Again I wondered, could my nail file do any damage? I pressed it into my own throat to find out.

I searched for my jugular with my right hand while sticking the point with my left. I steered with my knees.

Wait a minute. This isn't safe driving. If I puncture my throat, I'll end up in the ditch. I need to try this at home.

I wasn't laughing yet. But I would.

If you have been treated for recurrent major depression, you might see the runaway train approaching. I was a lamb in January 2005, a little lamb led to Prozac slaughter, soon to be followed by Celexa slaughter, Remeron slaughter, nortriptyline, Cymbalta, and Effexor (God help me) slaughter. I didn't know what a mistake they all would be. My doctor, a family physician, didn't know. But, following standard protocol (swing twice, then refer), she would soon bail and send me on to my first psychiatrist, let's call her The Newbie, to be followed by a series of psychiatrists who also didn't know but thought they did. They thought their pills held more magic than the family physician's pills (same pills) because they are, after all, psychiatrists.

If you have tried a number of antidepressants, if you dutifully "keep trying," if your depression keeps coming back, and it keeps getting worse, something has to give. More on that later.

Meanwhile, you could use a laugh.

That is why I wrote *Prozac Monologues.*

So I went off Prozac for none of the reasons I should have, like irritability, insomnia, physical agitation, and, oh yeah, bizarre thoughts, but for something more mundane: it gave me diarrhea. I had mentioned it to my doctor, but she thought the diarrhea was from stress and would resolve itself. Three weeks into it, I went online and discovered it was a side effect of Prozac. That's when I quit. All on my own. They don't like it when you do that.

On January 25, 2005, I boarded the plane for Costa Rica, my nail file hidden in my checked bag in case the TSA changed the rules that morning. Also, this nail file was making me nervous. What might it suggest I do next? *And would the TSA know?* I put a yellow legal pad and a ballpoint pen in my carry-on. I had an idea for a comedy routine and thought I might make some notes.

For the next eight days in Costa Rica, my wife, Helen, went to the beach, explored colorful barrios, visited my grandmother (yes, *my* grandmother), tasted new foods, and tried to lure me out with her reports of all her adventures. She told me about the *mercado,* a mere window on the front of a house, where she bought orange juice because she was dehydrated, the brilliant blue suddenly in front of her when she turned the corner to the beach, the child who offered to sell her the iguana he had killed with a machete. ("Does it taste like chicken?" she asked.) All the while, I wrote. And wrote. And wrote. When I filled up one side of the yellow legal pad, I wrote on the back. When I filled up the back, I wrote in the margins. When I filled up the margins, I wrote between the lines.

  * *Increase in goal-directed activity or psycho-motor agitation.*

That's one of the symptoms of bipolar disorder. Just four of those writing, writing, writing days would have ticked the Bipolar II box. I returned to Iowa with seven chapters. Two weeks later, the book was finished, nine monologues conceived as stand-up comedy routines with a hidden subtext: trying to figure out what had happened to my brain on Prozac, and why I had thought to put a nail file to my doctor's neck.

Where did that thought come from, to put a nail file to this woman's neck?

But it wasn't just a thought. I saw myself do it. What was it?

I had another appointment when I got home from Costa Rica to get a new antidepressant. I told my doctor about the book and writing maniacally every day of my vacation. The word "maniacally" raised a red flag. She screened for bipolar because people with bipolar disorder aren't supposed to take antidepressants. Antidepressants can make them crazy.

She asked, "Are you manic?"

I said what anybody who thought she was Jesus Christ come back as Jessica Christ might have said: "I'm not manic. I'm excited!"

  * *A distinct period of abnormally and persistently elevated, expansive, or irritable mood, lasting at least one week.*

That, my friends, is not *one* of the symptoms of bipolar. It is the *core* symptom.

She missed it. I was excited. She prescribed Celexa to replace the Prozac. And I was on my way to a whole new trip in February 2005. You would not like to have gone with me on this one.

After Celexa totally eliminated sleep from my life experience, the doctor referred me to a psychiatrist, the previously mentioned Newbie, who prescribed Remeron, and I was plunged into the depths of despair in March 2005. I quit that one too. In May I took myself to the rocky shores of Lake Superior for a solo retreat. When I wasn't climbing the rocks and reminding myself not to hurl my body off them, I worked my way through a book on dream interpretation, trying different techniques. It occurred to me to treat my rogue thought as a dream. A *waking* dream?

My therapist acquired after Costa Rica had been of no help whatsoever. Why put a nail file to my doctor's neck? She had been my doctor for over a decade, one of the most sought-after family practitioners in a university town filled with good doctors. We first met when she examined Jacob, my son from my starter marriage. She explained to this nervous eight-year-old that she would examine a sample of his rash to figure out what was causing it. He asked how she would get the sample. "I'll cut your arm off and put it under the microscope." After a beat, he decided she was alright. This was back before I had health insurance, and I only saw her for Jacob's medical emergencies. Adventurous sort, he had a few. I got my own physicals done at Lesbian Health Night at the free medical clinic. And there she was, doing volunteer physicals, as she did once a week every week on her day off, and did mine too.

But my therapist was convinced I must have been angry at this doc. I wracked my brain and dredged up every conceivable reason I might be angry at her. Well, once a few years back, she did make a mistake. She couldn't figure out what was making me sick and spent several weeks putting me through a boatload of tests. Then Helen went online and discovered my problem was a side effect from the medication I was taking for arthritis. But my doc apologized. I mean, really apologized, not one of those politician or malpractice lawyer apologies. She took responsibility for the error and explained how she would make amends. She would tell the story of her mistake to a class she was teaching that week, as a case study illustrating the need to pay attention to side effects. With such an apology, how could I stay angry? After weeks of exploring subconscious motivation with my therapist, there was never an "Aha!"

So on this dream retreat, treating the whole nail file experience as a waking dream, I had a conversation with each of the principals: myself, my doc, and the nail file itself. That was one of the techniques. That's when the nail file told me "the point," which was that I needed more and better treatment than I was getting.

A decade later, I would return to Costa Rica and pick up my original manuscript. It turns out to be a blazing case study for a different diagnosis: Bipolar II. I don't have the extreme mania to which my doc's question and my answer referred. That would be what you think bipolar means, wild and crazy, Bipolar I. Bipolar I is much more complex than *wild and crazy*, but the movies mostly show you people breaking things and driving their cars into rivers. That's why I denied being manic; I wasn't breaking things and was only *thinking* about driving my car into the river. Bipolar II also is more complex, but the behavior part isn't as dramatic. My therapist read the monologues hot off the episode, but she didn't see it either. If *some*body had seen it, if my nail file had told me the *real* point, that my diagnosis of major depression was wrong, and not only did I need more and better treatment, I needed *different* treatment, my life would be different today. What if. What if.

Whatever.

I love *Prozac Monologues,* those original monologues, with a mother's love. Even more, with an author's love. Sometimes I want to scream at the manuscript, shake it, and throw it against the wall. Then I long to be back at that place where it was possible to write a book in three weeks with sentences that go on for days and explore new paths and even whole barrios and circle round on themselves and tie themselves in a knot and stop just short of strangling themselves to death.

Examine the evidence yourself. Each of the original monologues is identified by the title *Prozac Monologues* and the date that I wrote it. It reflects the state of my addled brain *on that day*. Every now and then, my many-years-wiser self will interrupt those comedy routines with a chapter identified as *A Voice from the Edge*. Those chapters are about what I wish I had known a long time ago, the symptoms of mania and hypomania, research about the bipolar brain, and what recovery means on the bipolar spectrum.

It has been a long, strange trip. And yet the trip testifies to recovery. It wasn't what the original *Prozac Monologues* promised. It wasn't what Prozac promised, either. But recovery is still possible. I want you to know that.

That is why I wrote *Prozac Monologues: A Voice from the Edge.*

Prozac Monologues

Bizarre: In which I decide to write a book

Sunday, January 23, 2005

OK, let's start with the basic Prozac dilemma. Just who is the crazy one around here, anyway? If you get up in the morning happy, content, secure, at peace, ready to go out and carry on your activities of daily living, full of confidence and a sense of purpose, then tell me, are you pathologically delusional? Or are you on Prozac?

Citizens of the United States of America spend more on trash bags than the gross national product of ninety of the world's 130 nations. Stop right there. Think about that many trash bags. Think about all that trash! Who is the crazy one around here, anyway?

We get a sliver of time to enjoy our existence on this wildly extravagant planet, and we spend precious moments of it watching couples compete for cash prizes on the basis of how many maggots they can eat, until the maggot-eating is interrupted by somebody who wants to sell you an air freshener that uses electricity to circulate chemical compounds around your living room to make you think you are outdoors. According to this public service announcement of one more amazing American innovation, the fan is the latest advance in civilization that will enable you to stop feeding your shih tzu little treats, which you previously had to do to get him to wag his little tail to disperse the chemical compounds around your living room.

So now you take Prozac to get yourself up off the sofa where you have been sitting in a semi-catatonic state, watching the maggot-eating and dog-treating, out of your pajamas and into your four-wheel-drive SUV, which you were compelled to purchase after viewing those commercials of SUVs climbing over mountainous terrain beside raging rivers, but which you happen to use to commute an hour and forty-five minutes on some freeway to work in a cubicle with a picture of mountainous terrain and raging rivers and some motivational caption beneath, so you can buy the air freshener with its self-contained and electrically operated fan that disperses the chemicals that make you think that you are outdoors, because you wouldn't actually want to go outdoors, the air is so nasty from the fumes from your SUV. Who is the crazy one around here?

Don't even get me started on the taxes you will pay from your job in your cubicle to fund somebody's research into that missile that can shoot another missile out of the sky, which we need to protect ourselves from the bad guys who can bring down two one hundred–story buildings armed with the equivalent of a Swiss Army knife. If it's your job to figure out how to shoot that missile out of the sky, stop taking Prozac and find something else to do with your life. Or go back to your sofa. Please.

OK, now I'm starting to sound like Michael Moore. Maybe I need to take my Prozac. Let's just call this the Crazy Delusion, a concept not original to me, and of which you can think of your own examples, I don't need to continue this rant, which is not really the point but only its context.

In short, it's hard to know whether depression is a problem of distorted thinking or the consequence of clarity. In either case, sitting on the sofa in your pajamas does not turn the economic engine of this great nation, no matter what you are watching. With the exception of the pharmaceutical industry's economic engine. It's no skin off their nose that you are stuck on the sofa. They will keep making money as long as they are able to sell you images of people who are happy and confident, popping their Prozac, which you really start to believe while you are still sitting on that sofa, watching those images over and over and over again.

Have you noticed how all the ads for antidepressants run during the afternoon soaps? If you are not depressed, you probably haven't noticed, because you are out at work, turning that economic engine. Those pharmaceutical guys know where to find their audience, and when: on the sofa, in our pajamas, in the middle of the afternoon.

I am talking to you, the one in the pajamas. You thought you might get up and go for a walk, like you promised your sweetie, who has gone to work, that you would. But here it is, two o'clock in the afternoon. The recap of yesterday's episode comes on and before you manage to find the remote to turn it off after the last soap, that theme song begins. It sounds inspirational, but for some reason, you start to cry. After the theme song and before today's episode, it is time for that gentle, compassionate voice that lists all your symptoms, including another one that you have, now that the voice mentions it, but until now you didn't realize that it is on the list, so you must be even sicker than you thought. Who is that guy that understands you so well, better than your doctor, it seems, and therefore must know exactly what you need to ask your doctor to prescribe?

Do you think you are the only person on the planet stuck on the sofa? Twenty percent of the population of the United States will experience an episode of depression sometime over their lifetimes,[1] half of them a whole lot of episodes.[2] Half of that twenty percent are sometimes way up, but more often way down.[3] And another 1.5 percent feel lousy all the time.[4] You can figure in any given month that one in twenty people just feels like crap.

Wow. With so much company, how is it you feel this alone?

But there's good news! You don't have to feel like this! There is a little pill you can take. Half a dozen people come on after that gentle compassionate voice to tell you how it changed their lives. And it has a low risk of sexual side effects. Every single one of them, six in total, grinning from ear to ear and telling you the same thing, low risk of sexual side effects. Like you're worried about losing the active sex life you have been enjoying because you have all that energy stored up at the end of the day when you didn't manage to get out of your pajamas.

Now let's say your sweetie comes home and finds you still in your pajamas. Again. She or he is not as gentle and compassionate as that announcer. She used to be, but not anymore. She is fed up. She tells you that somebody at work takes this medication. And it has a low risk of sexual side effects. Or maybe not. That particular medication is relatively new, i.e., not available as a generic, and you can't afford it unless you have really good drug coverage. And what would the chances of that be, that the one who needs really good drug coverage actually has it? More likely, somebody at work is taking Prozac. Everybody and his mother-in-law and her rabbi are taking Prozac, which you don't know now, but you will find out if you start to admit to other people that you do, too, once you do. The thing is, it works. I mean, we're talking about somebody, your sweetie's coworker, that is, who is actually at work. In street clothes and everything. So, your sweetie has made an appointment for you to go see your doctor tomorrow.

Now, if you don't have a sweetie, or if yours isn't paying as close attention as mine is, or is not as well informed as mine is, then you will have to make the appointment yourself. Really, you have to. It's even more important than getting out of your pajamas. The doctor won't mind if you come to the appointment in your pajamas, as long as you get there. If the knife is already to your wrist, don't call for an appointment. Just dial 911. Somebody will come and give you a ride.

Once you get that one thing done, then you are on the road to recovery. It may turn out to be a long road. It may have many roundabout turns along the way. But you will pick up strength as you go. Really, you will.

At the point that you finally do get up off the sofa, then you have a choice to make. You can rejoin the Crazy Delusion. Or you can participate in it just enough—because complete avoidance is impossible—that sofa sitting is one more variation of the delusion . . . Where was I? Oh yeah, just enough to *resist* the delusion, to do your part to make the world a little less crazy, to care, to walk, to love, to learn, to touch, to live. You might have to get better before you get good at all those things. But then choose your direction. Take Prozac if it helps you *to live*. But I can't bring myself to recommend it so you can feel OK about being as crazy as the rest of the world.

Now. All of the above is still the context in which we must consider the meaning of the word "bizarre."

Consider: bizarre is good, when we're talking about the movie *Fargo*. Unless you didn't like *Fargo*, in which case possibly you consider bizarre to be bad when talking about any subject.

But even if you liked the movie *Fargo*, bizarre is bad when we are talking about Prozac. For all the good that Prozac is doing for your neighbor, your secretary, your mother-in-law, your bus driver, and your child's soccer coach, every once in a while there's this problem. It's a side effect called "bizarre thoughts."

If you start having "bizarre thoughts" while on Prozac, it is bad. Seriously, you need to tell your doctor. Some people, not many but some, have gotten into serious trouble when Prozac induced bizarre thoughts. More on that later.

When it occurs to you that your brain is about to explode, how do you know whether what you're experiencing is good bizarre or bad bizarre? And now that you have been exposed to *my* thinking for the last few pages, do you trust me to tell you?

True confessions: I have been off Prozac for fourteen days, cold turkey. I am writing as fast as I can, because my thoughts are getting less bizarre. But they seem desperately important. I want to get them down before I lose them.

So here goes: bad bizarre thoughts are the sort that scare the person who is having them and make you afraid to tell your doctor or your sweetie about them. Those are the bizarre thoughts you absolutely *must* tell your doctor and your sweetie about.

Suck it up, or you could end up, well, like me. Remember, after telling the doctor about the bizarre thoughts and after getting help, if either of us decides that trying to survive wasn't such a great idea, or is just too damn much work after all, we can always stop trying. How's that for bizarre.

Good bizarre thoughts, on the other hand, are the kind you can turn into a movie or book or reality show and make money. Those you should copyright.

Notice that "good" does not mean the same thing as "beneficial," except in the monetary sense, which at least is something. For that matter, "bad" does not mean the same thing as "*not* beneficial," since bad bizarre thoughts do give you useful information, if you are able to use it, which is that you need a different medication.

Can you anticipate the runaway train fast approaching on the horizon? I did get up off the sofa, out of my pajamas, and into the doctor's office. I did go on Prozac and eagerly anticipated the fulfillment of my pharmacological quest for happiness, contentment, security, peace, once more being able to get up, go out, and carry on my activities of daily living, full of confidence and a sense of purpose. After two months of vastly different results, there came that critical doctor's appointment when we decided to increase my dose. I can't remember the vague things I said to my doctor about poor concentration that led her to decide I wasn't taking enough Prozac. But I remember quite clearly what I did *not* tell her, that as I walked into the office, I had this image of me sticking the point of my nail file into her neck.

By the end of this image, a whole sequence, really, playing itself out in my head like a movie that reaches out and grabs the channel-surfer who never made any kind of conscious decision to stop in front of it, I saw myself being escorted by two burly male nurses upstairs. My doctor's office is in the hospital. The psych ward is one floor up. Convenient.

If I were on the psych ward, I would have missed an upcoming meeting at church, in fact, the Annual Meeting. Which is why I decided I would not stick a nail file in my doctor's neck, so I would not miss the Annual Meeting.

Plus, I bet she could take me.

The phrase "a danger to oneself or others" came to mind. And I didn't like that thought at all. So I decided, in addition to the decision not to stick a nail file into her neck, which was a good decision, that I also would not tell her it had occurred to me to do it, lest she decide that not having done it was a technicality, though an important technicality from both our points of view, and she would have me escorted upstairs to the psych ward anyway. Instead, we mutually decided that I needed more Prozac.

That was a bad decision, one I am not qualified to make, even when my brain is not being chemically scrambled. And in my freaked-out incompetence, I was not able to give information to the person who *is* competent to make the decision, which is how I got more Prozac, which led to more bizarre thoughts. Bad bizarre thoughts.

Now, bad bizarre thoughts are not necessarily fatal. They give your caretakers useful information, once you tell them about them. It took about four days before I confessed to Helen, who's getting a crash course in those words she said nine years ago, *for better, for worse.* I haven't told my doctor yet, not the precise details that would concern her most directly. I plan to tell her at my appointment when I get home from Costa Rica. About bizarre thoughts in general, that is. I still plan to be sketchy about the details, such as the identity of the person into whose neck I imagined myself sticking my nail file. Actually, I don't think I'll mention the nail file at all, because she might wonder if I have it on my person at the time and that might make her nervous.

Ultimately, the difference between bad bizarre thoughts and good bizarre thoughts comes down to one switch. It's not the money switch, though the money could factor in. If you have bad bizarre thoughts, the money is flowing *away* from you in the form of co-pays. If you have good bizarre thoughts, the money is flowing *toward* you in the form of royalties. But money is the bottom line much less often than we think. Calling it the bottom line is another part of the Crazy Delusion. And money is not the switch of which I now speak. The real switch is the healing switch. It switches when you laugh.

And eventually, that is how this story ends. At least, for today. After I was off Prozac about a week, I started to laugh. After two weeks, Helen can laugh, too—maybe now that my laughter has stopped sounding like that creepy Peter Lorre laugh. She even pointed out the *really* bizarre part of this story. Remember the meeting at church I would have missed if I had stuck a nail file in my doctor's neck? The Annual Meeting—every person at that meeting, and me, too, if I had been thinking clearly at the time, would have paid big bucks, full fee, not just the co-pay, to get a doctor's note to miss that particular Annual Meeting.

Which is funny, when you think about it. And when you are recovering from Prozac.

A Voice from the Edge

Flight

---

* Flight of ideas or subjective experience that thoughts are racing.

I have a new doctor now.

The doctor into whose neck I did not press my nail file retired, and what could I do? I left Iowa in 2012 and moved to Central Oregon. Well, that wasn't the only reason I moved, but it made me think I might as well. I was in my Oregon doctor's office in January 2015 to ask about trying another mood stabilizer. Many years after Prozac I am still on my pharmacological quest for happiness, contentment, security, etc., but I don't do antidepressants anymore. Now we are searching a different class of meds, a whole new shelf.

Once you step into bipolar land and say the word out loud, you notice a little freeze in the person to whom you said it. But my new doctor is cool. He doesn't seem freaked out at all about my new diagnosis. He encouraged me to try the mood stabilizer. It was the last one on the mood stabilizer shelf, so this stage of the quest was winding down. Then he gave me some feedback. He said my thoughts were not as organized as they had been on previous visits.

I told him I was planning a seven-course meal with wine pairings for the premiere of the new *Downton Abbey* season.

That's when his eyes glazed over. I could guess the note he was making: "flight of ideas."

But it wasn't a change of topic. I knew the connection between my "not as organized" thoughts and *Downton Abbey*. I was explaining the circumstance that had made me a little excited lately, acknowledging insight into my scattered thoughts. No, not quite manic, more like excited. Wouldn't you be excited if you were planning a seven-course meal with wine pairings?

But the appointment had already run long, it wouldn't change the outcome, and—whatever—I let him make his note.

Collective nouns: pride of lions, fleet of ships, host of angels. Flight of ideas. Isn't that what ideas are supposed to do—fly? Most closely related to that host of angels, I think.

Mosby's Medical Dictionary defines flight of ideas as "a continuous stream of talk in which the patient switches rapidly from one topic to another and each subject is incoherent and unrelated to the preceding one or is stimulated by some environmental circumstance."

Remember the sofa / reality TV / air fresheners / shih tzu / SUV / inspirational posters / air pollution / taxes / 9/11 thing from my "Bizarre" monologue? Well, it could be a writer's choice of style. On the other hand, it could be the literary expression of a brain wave that goes on for days and explores new paths and even whole barrios and circles back on itself and ties itself in a knot and stops only if somebody hits me on the head with a two by four.

Or lithium.

I think Mosby just can't keep up.

See, the medical world thinks that flight of ideas is a sign of mania or hypomania (mania-lite), the so-called "up" part of bipolar, a symptom of a state that comes and goes. Those of us who occasionally experience mania or hypomania know differently.

For people with bipolar, flight of ideas is not part of the transient state of mania. It is an enduring trait. Our brains are wired with the capacity to manage a whole lot more connections than our psychiatrists can manage. They are plodding along from A to B to C, taking their own sweet neuro-*normal* time while we have skipped over LMNOP, which we do know are there, yes, we do, but we, like Dr. Seuss, are more interested in what is on beyond Z. Like how the monologue began on the sofa, paused at air fresheners, zipped over to SUVs and ended up at 9/11, all in one nonstop flight.

The process of labeling says as much about the psychiatrist as it does about the patient, as do most diagnostic criteria. Think of Mosby. Nevertheless, flight of ideas is a telling symptom, because when we are balanced, we know better than to leap ahead of our psychiatrists, at least out loud, and we control our impulses to do so. So they never know. When we are manic, it's not our ideas over which we lose control. It's our impulses. When we let fly in front of our doctors, we are not in our balanced and buttoned-down state. That is when they increase our dose.

Now back to *Prozac Monologues,* back to 2005. After our flight to Costa Rica, there I was, still flying . . .

Prozac Monologues

No Sense of Humor: In which my doctor does not smile

Tuesday, January 25, 2005

They say laughter is the best medicine. But don't try your material out on your doctor. Doctors have no sense of humor.

Or at least they don't seem to laugh at bizarre thoughts. Is it because if you laugh yourself well, they can't bill the insurance company? No—I take it back. Cheap shot. I am not accusing them of not having your best interest at heart. Not at all. When it comes to depression, I think that your best interest and the doctor's truest intention are in perfect alignment. I really do. On the other hand, no comment about the pharmaceutical companies' intentions.

No, this lack of sense of humor seems almost congenital. You can hardly get a doctor to crack a smile, even when your diagnosis is warts. Well, OK, they smile when the news is good. That's not the same as humor. Then, for all you know, they're merely pleased with themselves. The shadow on Mama's mammogram was not cancer after all, and her doc acts like it's on account of his brilliance. If he were so brilliant, why did he have her planning her funeral over the weekend while she waited for the follow-up test results? But if the news is good, she's pleased too. Why quibble?

If the news is good, then you don't need any better medicine than what you have already received. Focus, Goodfellow, focus.

If laughter is the best medicine and doctors have no sense of humor, then you understand the meaning of the saying, "Physician, heal thyself." I wonder where the saying came from. It's in the Bible—did you know? But it was already a saying before it got to the Bible. In Luke, Jesus says, "Doubtless you will quote to me this proverb, 'Physician, heal thyself'" (Luke 4:23, English Standard Version). Where did Jesus hear the proverb? It's not in the Book of Proverbs. Maybe, since Luke is the only gospel that records it, it actually was Luke who knew the proverb, because somebody quoted it to him, on account of how he was supposed to have been a physician.

I think Luke had a sense of humor. The story about how Jesus healed the Gerasene demoniac by sending his legion of demons into a herd of swine that proceeded to jump over a cliff, so the neighbors asked Jesus to leave town before he bankrupted them (I'm not kidding—read Luke 8) could be an ironic commentary on the Crazy Delusion. Well, you have to have a sense of humor yourself to imagine an evangelist making an ironic commentary on the Crazy Delusion. But maybe Luke developed his sense of humor after he started traveling with Paul. Paul is a lot easier to take, if taken with a sense of humor, let me tell you, in case you haven't read Paul yourself.

In case you are a physician, or somebody who may have a sense of humor, but not of the ironic sort, let me explain what this saying, "Physician, heal thyself," means. It is a rebuke. It is said to people who cannot do for themselves what they purport to do for others.

You could say it to a physician who smokes, if you are of a literal mind. Or you could say it to a family therapist who is getting a divorce. But don't. That poor soul has enough trouble already. Or else is unable to benefit from your insight into his/her situation, either because he/she isn't particularly receptive to anybody's insight, which might explain the divorce, or maybe because you're a jerk. It's hard to benefit from the insight of a jerk, even if it's good insight.

You might also say the phrase "Physician, heal thyself" to people who call themselves Christian, who seem so preoccupied with the state of your soul that they have no discernible time to be concerned with the state of their own. That's not a jab at Christians in general. I am one myself, which is how I know this obsession with other people's behavior is incredibly ironic, not to mention bizarre, even if it seems to be common these days. And it gives Jesus a bad name to boot. You'd think they would want to avoid doing that.

However, in my experience, even non-Christians, or rather, especially non-Christians can figure out the difference between Jesus and that kind of Christian. My real complaint is that they give the rest of us Christians a bad name.

Do you remember after 9/11 when they said irony was dead? Boy, am I glad that didn't last, or I'd be dead too.

But not doctors. The death of irony didn't touch them because doctors are not ironic to begin with. My point, and I do have one, about the "Physician, heal thyself" thing—if they can't laugh, they are missing a significant tool for self-healing. So they might not be able to do for themselves what they purport to do for others. Remember, humor is what triggers the healing switch.

But I don't think I ever got a call from the doctor's office saying the doctor had to cancel my appointment because the *doctor* was sick. Now that is amazing, and clearly a demonstration of enormous powers of self-healing. I mean, have you ever thought about what goes on in a typical doctor's day? Besides it being long, I mean. Think about a workday that starts with hospital rounds at six, before their patients are even up, or at least care to be up. No, let's skip the details—which you won't often catch me deciding to do.

Nevertheless, it does occur to me, when I am healthy and not actually in the doctor's office—like, when it's not about me—that right before she comes in to see me, she could have been looking at a nasty rash. The kind you don't want to touch. Maybe in a place you really don't want to show anybody anyway, much less explain how you got it. But the doctor has to look at it, and worse, has to listen to the explanation, and even worse, has to ask for the explanation. Then the doctor has to figure out how much of what she has heard actually are the facts of the matter. Then she has to wash her hands, which I am exceedingly glad that she does, and come deal with me, poor soul (her, not me, in this case), and try to read my mind, which is full of thoughts, the details of which she would not want to ponder if she knew what they were.

I wonder if that's why she didn't actually ask what was on my mind that "bizarre thought" day. When she repeated the perfectly good recommendation that she gave me the previous appointment—"Go talk to a therapist, already!"—that I didn't follow originally and was vague about then, because I am still hoping for the fulfillment of my pharmacological quest for well-being, since taking a pill every night is much less embarrassing than telling another living soul what is going on inside my bizarre little brain, poor soul (me this time), I tried to distract her with an entirely new ailment I couldn't quite describe or remember how long I've had, or what makes it worse, and I didn't even mention until her hand was on the doorknob to go out the door to the next appointment, who was probably going to cough all over her.

I have a physician friend who tells me that when she has run out of patience with uncommunicative or rambling or downright deceptive patients, and she wants to get to the heart of the matter, she stands up and puts her hand on the doorknob. That's when the real stuff gets said. But my doctor, when she puts her hand on the doorknob, simply turns it and leaves. Clearly, my last-minute rush of words wasn't compelling enough to turn her around. What do you think—if I mentioned the nail file when her hand was on the doorknob, would she have come back in or kept heading out?

Two thoughts occur to me. First, how come she's never sick? And second, how does she survive dealing with sick people all day long if she has no sense of humor? Is she on Prozac?

I'm not going to survive dealing with myself without a sense of humor. How many of me does a doctor have to survive every day?

I decided that it is my responsibility to solve the mystery of the doctor's missing sense of humor. I played hours of FreeCell, which is what I do lately when I am searching for the next six words in a writing project, until the answer came to me. Here it is. Humor is a boundary doctors are trained not to cross with their patients.

I don't know why it is a boundary. I didn't take that class. I didn't even go to medical school. It is a conclusion drawn from my own experience. I did go to seminary to become a priest. Did I mention I am a priest, an ordained minister in the Episcopal Church? A priest forever after the order of Melchizedek—that's what it says on the certificate. We get depression too. Isn't that a bite.

Melchizedek was a random priest who made a cameo appearance in the book of Genesis, took an offering from Abraham, and was never seen again. I wonder if he had depression. Does it go with the job? Once I was at a continuing education day for clergy on the topic of depression. My discussion table didn't want to discuss the questions. Instead, we compared our meds.

Clergy have our own boundaries. Humor is not one of them, except for certain kinds of humor, though not irony, lucky for me.

Here is my definition. A professional boundary is a line that, if the professional crosses it, then the professional/client relationship changes in such a way that the professional is no longer able to give the help that the client came to the professional to receive. The success of the giving and receiving of help is dependent on maintaining the helper/helped relationship. That is why it doesn't work if your lawyer is your partner in crime, if your priest takes you to bed, or if your doctor laughs at your jokes.

How does humor interfere with the doctor/patient relationship, you ask? Remember the rash my doctor was hypothetically looking at before she came in to see me. Part of the doctor's job is to figure out how much of that poor soul's explanation represents the facts of the matter. That is part of almost any encounter between any doctor and patient, at least if the patient is conscious, lucid, and verbal, not like the diabetic German tourist who got his foot amputated in Costa Rica, much to his surprise when he regained consciousness, poor soul. He started out in a coma, so they had nothing to go on but the physical evidence. But if the patient can talk, then the doctor has to figure out the relationship between the words that come out of the patient's mouth and the actual facts of the matter.

If the doctor laughs at your jokes, it encourages you to invent more material, which adds to the difficulty of sorting through the words that come out of your mouth and the actual facts of the matter, not to mention gobbling up the valuable minutes the insurance company is willing to pay the doctor to figure you out.

Now, doctors and anybody else who lives or works around them may well protest that doctors have a great sense of humor and tell the wildest jokes, though not always in good taste. (I don't think good taste is a requirement for the "laughter is the best medicine" thing.) But they don't do it around their patients. Think *Scrubs*, that sitcom about medical residents. Think *M*A*S*H*. I will not only grant the point, but I will commend it. And now I do revise my opening claim to insert the phrase "around their patients." Doctors have no sense of humor *around their patients*. There. Are you satisfied?

I don't mind that doctors have a sense of humor they reveal only to their friends and family and coworkers. I don't even mind if their sense of humor is a little bizarre, if *Scrubs* and *M*A*S*H* are any indication. After all, laughter is the best medicine, and I'm glad my doctor is not sick. Because I am, and I need another appointment when I get home from Costa Rica.

Only it's a little disconcerting when I say my diarrhea has improved to the "soft-ball stage" (like in fudge-making) and my doctor gets a pained look on her face, as if when she figures out the relationship between the words that came out of my mouth and the actual facts of the matter, she concludes that I am dying inside. I really wanted her to smile. Instead, she gave me "The Look."

A Voice from the Edge

Squirrel!

Attention too easily drawn to unimportant or irrelevant external stimuli.

Back to life in the United States, where a decade later, the issues remain remarkably the same.

I get up from my laptop to get a glass of water, and there is the pork chop that needs defrosting for lunch. Next to the microwave is the grocery list, including the vegetables for lunch. On the way to my wallet, I see laundry to be folded. On a shelf in the linen closet are my empty pill cases. On the counter where I carry the pill cases and the pills to fill them is the pork chop that still needs to be defrosted for lunch.

Sometimes I wander in a circle chanting, "Finish something, finish something, anything, finish something."

Like that Tuesday, January 25, 2005, when I was thinking about the doctor who didn't laugh. On the way I wandered past insurance companies, Mama's mammogram, biblical exegesis, and a nasty rash. Finally, the doctor! But no, it was a different doctor. Two wrong doctors and some Costa Rican surgeons. Then the doctor who didn't laugh.

Distractibility. To be precise, from the big book of diagnoses, the *Diagnostic and Statistical Manual of Mental Disorders*
(DSM): *attention too easily drawn to unimportant or irrelevant
external stimuli.*

Is that how the diabetic German tourist got in there? I think
I overheard somebody reading the *Tico Times* at breakfast. Helen
said, "You're *not* going to write about the diabetic German tourist,
are you?"

Was he an *irrelevant external stimulus*? I thought he added
local color. Who gets to say what is irrelevant? According to the
DSM, the one making the diagnosis.

Finish something, finish something . . .

Prozac Monologues

The Look: In which she saves my life anyway

Wednesday, January 26, 2005

Depression is not an easy topic to discuss. I mean, it's so depressing. And when you've got it, you've got it for a long time and you think about it a lot. Pretty much all the time, in fact, even when you really want to be thinking about something else, like Costa Rica. Hence, even though it is compelling, it is, at the same time, boring. And when you are compelled to think a lot for a long time about a topic that is flat-out boring, it is, well, what else can I call it, depressing.

The fact that depression is boring has many ramifications, some of which impinge on the doctor/patient relationship and consequently on the difficulty of the doctor's task to determine the relationship between the words that come out of the patient's mouth and the actual facts of the matter, and as a consequence of that difficulty, the quality of the care received.

The alarm clock birds in the tree outside our window have gone off, 4:15 a.m., right on time. I don't know what kind of birds they are. I suppose I could get out of bed and look. But I am busy. Anyway, whatever they are, they are not songbirds. They make an ungodly racket, and wake up Helen, who has caught me already propped up in bed with my yellow pad, waxing multisyllabic. She's not crazy about all this time I am spending with my yellow pad. She wants me to go out with her today, to show me some surprise. Can't she see I'm busy? It's 4:15 a.m. and I am already multisyllabic.

When I write sermons, I check my "Flesch-Kincaid Grade Level" in the grammar check. It tells you how smart (or at least how educated) you have to be in order to understand a passage. Who knows if the Flesch-Kincaid thing means anything really, beyond telling me my words have a lot of syllables and my sentences are too long. If a preacher can't deliver the Good News without using big words and long sentences, I suspect the preacher is hiding something. There he is in the pulpit, reading his dissertation on a comparison of the soteriologies of the synoptic gospels, with no idea what it has to do with him, let alone his congregation.

4:15 a.m., am I already hiding something?

I wonder if there is a computer program to measure how far somebody's mind would have to bend to understand my uncharacteristically big words this morning. In the absence of the Word from on High (would that be Microsoft?) I make my own determination. I am writing at a 27 percent bent level.

You have never heard of the Bent Scale? Here is how it works: baseline 0 percent bent is a computer manual written by a native English-speaking engineer with no sense of humor, at least no sense of humor that the people who need the manual are able to discern. For all we know, computer manuals could be seriously bent, written by engineers who entertain themselves by messing with our minds. If the same manual is written in Japanese and then translated into English by somebody working in a cubicle in Mumbai, it is 8 percent bent. *Scrubs* comes in at 23 percent, *Twin Peaks,* a show from the early 1990s, at 38 percent.

Notice where I am positioning myself, farther out than *Scrubs*, but not as mean as *Twin Peaks*. As you approach 45 percent, you are in the personality disorder range. Above that, you start working your way into the functional schizophrenic to raging psychotic levels.

That gives you an idea of the possibilities for the Bent Scale. For all I know, this scale already exists in much greater detail and standardization of application. But I have never heard of it, because only doctors and therapists know about it, and to tell me about it would be a boundary violation. Or maybe it would make them feel uncomfortable to admit they can put a number, and in fact already *have* put a number to my suffering. So they call it a boundary violation and keep their secrets to themselves.

Those of you who have been in therapy, don't you always suspect as much? When you discover the person you have been talking to at a party and trying to impress with your sense of humor turns out to be a therapist—don't you suspect the therapist has already, on the basis of your fifteen minutes of witty conversation, assigned a number to you from the Bent Scale?

Do you want to know what your number is? I do. It might be fun to speculate on other partygoers' numbers. But no, that would feel like measuring other people's suffering, and it would make me feel depressed. Like I wasn't going to feel depressed at the end of a party, anyway.

But what is my number from these current musings? I rated myself a twenty-seven. If there really is a standardized Bent Scale out there, I hope somebody will tell me what my number is. Any chance they can get it into the grammar check on Word?

I wonder if my multisyllabic musings are an avoidance mechanism. Like humor, they support a certain emotional distance from my depression to enable me to analyze and document it without succumbing to it. See, I am doing it again.

But that's the thing. Depression is so depressing. And you can't get help unless you talk about it. And if you talk about it, you get more depressed. I can be having a perfectly delightful day—I am in Costa Rica, for goodness' sake! Then when I go to bed, I remember I have depression, and I start to cry. Bummer.

Some doctors learn to recognize avoidance mechanisms, such as humor and pseudo-intellectualism and multisyllabic speech, to get to what is being avoided, which would be the emotional reality behind all the clever speech. Clearly the doctor who failed to smile when I compared my stools to fudge-making is good at recognizing avoidance mechanisms. That is why I was busted.

The doctor who busted me and gave me The Look isn't really my doctor. She is somebody I went to see after I was so freaked out by the nail file in the neck thing that I was too freaked out to tell my real doctor about it. Which interfered with the quality of care my doctor was able to give me.

I was in a state. My real doctor thought I needed to spend a week in Costa Rica. Honest to God—that was her professional medical opinion. I have the email.

I decided to see another doctor. Actually, on the day in question, Helen refused to go to work and let me wring my hands in peace (is hand-wringing a side effect of Prozac?) until I made the appointment, because I had had the runs for three weeks, and she thought it was really stupid to bring the runs into a Central American country. She didn't want to worry about my electrolyte levels, even though Mama assured us there is an awfully nice doctor here in Costa Rica who speaks English and makes house calls, and even if my grandmother (did I mention my grandmother lives in Costa Rica?) does drink water straight from the tap and even with ice in it with no ill effects at all. In fact, she just celebrated her ninety-third birthday.

We didn't know it for sure yet, though we had been told. About the water, I mean. I knew that Grandma is ninety-three years old. We had to see it for ourselves. See, Helen has had prior emergency experience with dehydration in Mexico City. Truth be told, *she* was in a state. She insists she was not in a state. She was simply determined. A week ago, the Monday before our trip to Costa Rica, I was dealing with side effects from Prozac, side effects from sudden withdrawal from Prozac, and the original condition for which I had been prescribed Prozac, not to mention the runs. I was in no state to handle her state, which I still say she was in. Anyway, I agreed to go see the other doctor.

I knew the other doctor really does have a sense of humor, because I met her last month at a Christmas party. My problems with Prozac had already begun, but I didn't know it at the time. She had a sense of humor at the party. Something about cheesecake, I recall. She was in her kitchen, about to carve her standing rib roast, and telling us about the dessert, though I don't recall what about the cheesecake was so funny.

You really don't want to run into your doctor at parties and wonder if the doctor is trying to figure out the facts of the matter based on how your behavior at parties compares to the words that come out of your mouth at the office. My guess is the doctor doesn't want to be figuring out the facts of the matter either. She is at a party, for goodness' sake! I know this because when people meet me at parties and find out I am a priest, suddenly I am no longer at a party—I am At Work. Here I am, quietly trying to suck down my martini, while they explain to me that they are spiritual but not religious. I didn't ask!

No, save your party-going-with-doctors for other doctors, not your own. Then you can ask them for a second opinion.

So I made an appointment to get a second opinion about my state. Because it was my first appointment with this second doctor, it was a new patient appointment. Now, as I said, I was not really a new patient. I was more of a drive-by patient. But we hadn't talked about that yet. And besides, to give her any shot at figuring out the facts of the matter, she was going to have to (a) take my history, and (b) talk with me for an extended period of time. I don't think the health insurance companies code for "drive-by patient appointment." "New patient" has to cover it.

The second doctor's reception area was a far cry from my own doctor's hostile surroundings. The receptionist smiled, the chairs were comfortable, the plants were real, there was no psych ward hovering overhead. Before I could pick up a magazine, which was not torn, somebody handed me a patient history form.

You really do have to be patient to deal with all the patient history forms you will ever fill out, unless you can figure out how to see only one doctor in your adult lifetime, at least until you are no longer conscious, lucid, and verbal, and somebody else has to fill out the forms for you. Once I filled out a patient history form for my mother, when she was on oxycodone. It was interesting what she chose not to disclose.

The hardest part of the form is the family history. I can never remember whether my mother had cervical cancer or uterine cancer. The subject of diabetes has never arisen in conversations with my brothers. And Grandma has always been a little vague about her ailments. It is none of my business, really, much less my doctor's, from my grandma's point of view. All she wants is for people to know she *has* ailments, so they will take care of her.

I come from a long line of non-disclosers.

Then there is the page full of the patient's history, existing conditions and current symptoms. Now I do remember these, if you ask about them one at a time. I can tell you with absolute confidence right this exact minute that I have never had tuberculosis. But when whipping down a list of forty items, I run into "gallbladder," and I get confused. Are they asking if I have a gallbladder? Do I? What is "gallbladder," anyway? I remember back when I was a college sophomore and in the hospital for an appendectomy that the person in the next bed was there for "gallbladder." When the resident tried to stick a tube up her nose, she grabbed his tie and nearly strangled him to death. If you have ever had an NG tube inserted while you were conscious, you know this behavior on her part was not Prozac-induced; Prozac had not yet been invented. It wasn't even bizarre. It was self-de-fense. But no, they just took my appendix, not my gallbladder.

I did not get through the list before my name was called.

The big-ticket items were hiding at the bottom of the first column. There was no point in having come to this office unless I was going to fully disclose. Besides, Helen was looking over my shoulder. I circled everything.

It's funny, isn't it, how the mind works? If I was looking at a piece of paper, I was perfectly comfortable with words I couldn't say to the face of my fabulous doctor who has given me, what, eight pap smears, maybe ten, words like "suicidal thoughts" and "thoughts about hurting oneself or others."

We had a nice long chat, this drive-by doctor and I, about all the reasons I might have the runs and all the tests she would run to get the facts of the matter, though she did agree with my real doctor's evaluation and course of action, or rather inaction, that all the tests would be negative, and they would go away on their own after a week in Costa Rica. Nevertheless, she ordered a battery of tests she would not normally have run this soon in the course of this particular symptom, which is what I wanted, because this really was more about my "state" than about the runs, even though after eighteen days, the runs were indeed con-tributing to my state, which was reason enough to be rid of them.

Health insurance companies want doctors to do less testing and give only the tests and treatments directly indicated by the computer-generated protocol for the symptoms, which makes sense, I admit, on some level. Except doctors are not primarily technicians administering procedures according to particular protocols. That is just the way the insurance companies deal with them, assigning numbers to the sufferings of their custom-ers, and asking doctors to do the same.

But at the heart of the matter, doctors are healers. Really, for the most part, the body heals itself. But the doctor/patient relationship helps the patient's body get redirected when it is stuck in destructive instead of healing patterns. And the doctor needs flexibility to adjust the treatment according to what is going on in the relationship. Plus another five minutes.

That is why I needed to go to the second doctor, so I could get a new patient code, which would accommodate the extra five minutes.

When the doctor looked at the piece of paper with all those words circled on it, she didn't smile at my weak attempt at humor. Oh well. What she was most concerned about for my trip to Costa Rica was how I would manage my depression as the Prozac was leaving my system—which I could tell it was, because the dark suffocating cloud was coming back.

And now we had arrived at the heart of the matter. I knew this part. I could have conducted it myself. I *have* conducted it myself, when sitting across from some other poor soul in my own office. Did I have a "plan"? Well yes, I had a "plan." But I didn't "plan" to use my "plan." She didn't think that was funny either. In which case, there was no way I was going to tell her about the nail file.

I told her I felt more in control of my bizarre thoughts, less afraid of them, since I was learning to laugh at them, which was true. Actually, I had already started working on a comedy routine called "Bizarre" in my head. But I didn't tell her that, because there was no humor in sight. And she was working up to it. I could tell. Her face was rearranging itself into The Look.

She said, "Can you promise me you will not hurt yourself?"

Those are the words, spoken in a soft, low tone, that go with The Look. The Look is given with the chin down, looking up at you but straight in your eyes, this puppy dog kind of expression, as if to say, "It would hurt my feelings so very badly if you broke your promise to me." Some people are better at it than others. But she was fabulous. It was a sight to behold.

Now I know the lines. I have said them on occasion to another poor soul, trying to cover the time between the appointment with me and the next appointment with somebody who could offer more expert help. But I don't know how good I am at The Look myself. I have never practiced in front of the mirror. Good enough, I guess. Because I have never lost anybody.

Wow. What a concept. I have never lost anybody. It really isn't funny, is it, that responsibility.

Because I myself have given as well as received The Look, I noticed the technique. That is how I knew she was reaching deep beyond the technician of the best practices procedure, even beyond the healer, right into the heart of the witch doctor. She was casting a spell. And even though I noticed the technique, I deeply wanted this spell to work. This spell was truly in my best interest. It could save my life. So I looked into her eyes, took a deep breath, and let myself fall under the spell. Yes, I promise. I will not hurt myself.

Of course, behind the puppy dog in The Look is The Steel Trap, with its unspoken words, "You will not leave this office unescorted unless you can make this promise." And there is the safety net, in case you need to fall.

There is no insurance code for The Look. It is possible for the doctor to ask the questions and check them on a form and fill out the paperwork and never enter the sacred space that is crossed by means of The Look.

By the way, it isn't the promise that saves lives. Those are words out of a book. People lie if they don't care about the person who wants them to promise, or if they think the person asking doesn't care, or if they think they need to. Because, well, they need to.

No, it's the spell. The spell is cast by the willingness of the doctor to cross into that dark and sacred space. The person on whom the spell is cast discovers there is another human being on this planet who is willing to look deep into the pain, to acknowledge the danger there, to refuse to hide from it with intellectualism or humor or anything else, and to hand over a piece of his/her will to live.

If somebody gives you The Look, look back. Look deep. Allow that transfer of will to take place.

Say "Yes," if you mean it. Say "No," if you need more help right now.

And live.

A Voice from the Edge

Pressure

---

* More talkative than usual or pressure to keep talking.

Whew!

It wasn't your typical week in paradise. My brain ran like an eighteen-wheeler coming out of the Rockies with tumbling words and burning brakes until I could find the off ramp and slow my runaway brain by downshifting my mood.

Think Robin Williams. Now there was a guy who could talk. People use the word "manic" to describe his performances. Let's be clear. Williams acknowledged his recurrent depression, to which some doctors give the diagnosis bipolar-*ish*. But the Genie in *Aladdin* may have been stage behavior, a comedian's choice of style, not necessarily a symptom. Let 'er rip, Robin.

Nevertheless, like that.

I still had to get down the mountain.

Prozac Monologues

Leaping Lizards: In tribute to John Steinbeck's turtle

Thursday, January 27, 2005

The Pato Loco is a boutique hotel, which in the trade is what you call a hotel with only a few rooms, which I didn't know until my mother started using the phrase in emails that I did not know what to make of, and I looked it up on what is now her website and saw for myself. To put those two words together, "her" and "website," seemed a bit of a leap, even for Mama, who is not known for sitting still. The woman does not sit down. Retired once from the Social Security Administration, retired a second time from owning and operating a small-town radio station, four months ago my blind, seventy-two-year-old mother joined my sister the Voodoo Princess and her consort, Richie, to buy the Pato Loco in Playas del Coco, Costa Rica. Now she intends to feed the world, one plate of pasta at a time.

Upon hearing about this purchase, my pharmacist asked, "Was she lucid at the time?" I told the story when he asked where I was going when I bought the chloroquine, though Mama checked around, and nobody around Coco ever remembers a case of malaria, but evidently the Centers for Disease Control in the United States of America remembers, and they recommend I take it, and in any case the Red Cross will not allow me to donate blood for a year after I get back.

My pharmacist wasn't crossing a professional boundary by making such a comment. He was operating out of the other half of a dual relationship with me. He is my friend as well as my pharmacist. When we see each other at church or at parties, he does not behave like my pharmacist at all. For example, he does not comment on my choice of beverage at parties in relation to my pharmacological quest. Not that there is usually much to comment upon. I did once try mixing Ambien and scotch, which the Ambien label says not to. Not at a party, but at home right at bedtime, after I told Helen what I was doing in case I stopped breathing or something, because I was desperate for some sleep. It turns out she did not need to stay awake all night, checking my breathing and fretting, since I discovered the combination did not enhance the sleep-inducing properties of Ambien as promised, just the dizzy-inducing properties of scotch, which I drank hardly any of anyhow. I felt seasick the whole night through and was wide-awake as ever to experience it. Now I know and won't do that again, and you know, too, and don't need to repeat the experiment, unless you happen to like feeling seasick, in which case you probably read those drug warning labels for ideas, not warnings. I do that sometimes.

Back to my pharmacist's question—my mother is not always lucid. Sometimes she leaps. Leapt into five marriages, she did, and took six kids along for the ride. Sometimes she twirls. However, she was in her right mind and perhaps in her best mind—she would say so—when she bought the Pato Loco.

A month after Mama moved to Costa Rica, Grandma did too. Someday I will write *The Book of Grandma*. It will be the history of the twentieth century in America, starting with a childhood in Drumright, Oklahoma, in 1911, tracing the great migration out of the Dust Bowl, the labor movement in the middle decades, and loving her grandchildren through all the cultural dislocations of the rest of it: the Peace Movement, the Women's Movement, divorces, conversions, AIDS, entrepreneurship, weird new reproductive strategies in racehorses, wars in the Middle East, and pharmacological quests. Would that be your version of the twentieth century? It is my grandmother's.

For sixty-nine years, Grandma was the dearly beloved of Grandpa, until he died and was no longer there to wait upon her hand and foot, pretending to dominate her, though anybody who ever paid a bit of attention knew it was the other way round. Today Grandma is the queen who reigns from her wheelchair over the family table. Same job, new location. It's ironic how much this woman has moved, who, unlike her daughter, has been perfectly delighted to remain seated for the greater part of her lifetime.

The previous owners of the Pato Loco have become friends with my mother and sister and join us at the family table. Patricia is Dutch but grew up in Rome and supplied the original recipes. Antonello is the Pato Loco himself. That was his nickname when he was an Italian baseball star. It means "crazy duck," and he looks exactly like the logo of the hotel: pointy head, wild feathery hair, waddle, and all. Mama and the Voodoo Princess are retaining the Italian part of the restaurant because that is their established niche in the economy of Playas del Coco, which can support a lot of Italian restaurants, since Italians have been buying up condos sight unseen from Milan and Venice. But Mama added an international angle and makes meatloaf for a weekly special. She also makes jambalaya, goulash, baklava, cabbage rolls (Croatian, not Polish—she can tell you the difference, should you ask, and she wants you to ask), and anything else her heart desires and that expatriates will flock to the place to eat, and if they don't we will have the leftovers for lunch. Leftovers are important. Mama is not willing to cook or do much of anything purely to meet her own personal needs. She would starve without leftovers.

Mama has been to a lot of cooking schools. I wish she could deduct the tuition now that she has an international restaurant. She wouldn't think of it. She takes bizarre pride in paying taxes. According to my brother Kirk, who keeps track of her money, a whole lot of her children's inheritance has gone to the United States Treasury instead of to us, where it purchased a number of things I probably wouldn't have.

Oh well. It wasn't really my inheritance anyway, only my potential inheritance. It was her money. It still is, and she is welcome to spend it any way she wants, though I wish she wouldn't make it so freely available to those who spend it trying to invent a rocket to shoot another rocket out of the sky, should the second rocket ever be sent into the sky in the first place, when my congressman has explained it would be ever so much easier to get it to the United States in the mail, and he is smart and knows about these things.

I would rather she spend her money for dinner at Monique and Andre's. They are a French-Canadian couple who have turned their dining room into a restaurant and serve extravagant seven-course meals with wine pairings twice a week in Liberia, the big city twenty miles to the east. They keep track of every menu they ever serve and every guest who enjoys it, so they never ever serve the same thing twice to the same person, except for Andre's signature hors d'oeuvres, shrimps decorated with wisps of dill and caviar, each little egg placed separately. Andre beams over his shrimps, standing at the table until you admire his art and then pop it into your mouth. Mama goes there for special occasions; she took us on Monday to celebrate our visit, and it is the highlight of Grandma's life. Grandma was raised a Baptist in Oklahoma and promised not to drink alcohol back before she even knew what it was. Well, she knew it was the devil's drink. But Andre serves her a sip of wine from each bottle at each course because don't you think ninety-three years is long enough to keep the Pledge?

Anyway, that's how I would prefer my mother to spend her money, instead of on rockets. I suspect Grandma agrees with me, though she does not express opinions about such matters, except by subtle changes in the shape of her lips. You have to pay attention. Grandpa did. Nevertheless, it is my mother's money.

The international part of Pato Loco's restaurant's menu is the daily special that changes according to whim, though the expats are insisting she make Monday a regular meatloaf night. That way they won't miss it. The Italian part is still the bulk of the menu, pasta with twenty different names, including one dish Helen and I tried to get them to rename because in Spanish it sounds rude. It does in Italian too. But the Voodoo Princess refuses to change the name because she sells a lot of it. Maybe the customers like to say the name.

The family table is the eighth table, separated from the rest on a little patio, outside the open-air walls and covered by a tin extension of the tile roof. It is the heart of the place, where Grandma tells her stories about how at Christmas I used to steal the Baby Jesus and hide him in my undershirt (I was a baby at the time, and evidently already bent, though she says cute, as in, "You was such a cute little thing!"), and the Voodoo Princess and I try to figure out how to get Mama to take an afternoon nap so she doesn't look like she's suffering, a tired grimace on her face, when she seats guests at dinner, and how to hire more staff, and what are the chances the bartender will show up for the grand opening of the newly built bar, and what is the backup plan when he doesn't.

Last night the Voodoo Princess filled in for the bartender, and I stood next to her at the till and made change in *colones* for two hours while a traveling minstrel played Irish music on his guitar. It was a grand grand opening, grand to watch the Voodoo Princess work her stuff, especially when she jumped up on top of the bar, swished her red skirts up around her knees, and announced that happy hour was over, drinks now at the regular price, stay as long as you like.

You should come. It's worth the trip to meet her. You can find pictures on the website of the Voodoo Princess's consort, Richie, holding up various fish he has caught. But not pictures of the Voodoo Princess herself, because she is the photographer. You have to come to Costa Rica to meet her in person. Happy hour is a good time to do that. She will be happy to see you, especially if you bring Cheetos (original style) from the States, but even if you do not, because it's not about her.

Grandma is perfectly content to sit at the family table the entire day, except for her naps. Near the table, the hibiscus hedge is home to an assortment of butterflies who summer in the States, hovering around the sedum in my Iowa garden. I used to think they lived in the States and wintered in Costa Rica. Now I know better. They clearly belong here.

The rooster and a couple hens peck around in the shade of the hibiscus. These creatures are visitors; they don't belong to the hotel. If they did, Mama, child of the Great Depression, would be testing the hens to determine whether they are still laying, thereby paying their way. And if not, the daily special might be chicken and dumplings—a fabulous dish when Mama makes it. Don't even think of buying it in a can. It is a sin to make food that bad, not to mention selling it to poor souls in need of comfort. As one of those poor souls, I can tell you, buying a can of chicken and dumplings is like looking for love in all the wrong places.

It's a regular avian concert around the family table. Grandma especially likes the mourning doves, maybe because she can identify them, or maybe because some of the others really do sound obnoxious, especially at 4:15 in the morning. Loudest damn birds on the planet. Another kind looks like a pennywhistle—iridescent blue-black and so skinny that when you look at it straight on, it almost disappears. It sounds like a pennywhistle, too.

I did go somewhere with Helen this morning, a nature walk where I found out the pennywhistle bird is a grackle. I'm not sure about that. Dr. Will, the veterinarian who moved here from Kentucky, was going by our description, not his own sighting, and it seems to me this bird is skinnier than a grackle. Then again, Costa Ricans generally are skinnier than Iowans. Maybe it works the same with grackles.

Grackle—what an odd name to give a bird that glows iridescent blue and makes such magic with its voice. Their stateside cousins did not inherit their charm.

Dr. Will told us there are 108 different species of bats in Costa Rica. Grizzled gray beard, sturdy staff in hand, he climbs the hills between Coco and Ocotal every morning, and you are welcome to go with him. He departs from Father Rooster Bar on the Ocotal beach at 6:30 a.m. Remember your hat, your walking shoes, your water bottle and binoculars. Forget your camera. You can't capture an experience on film. While you are trying to preserve the moment, inevitably you fail to experience part of the moment. Instead, you experience the anticipation of the loss of the moment. There's enough loss in life already, let me tell you, no need to anticipate any. Unless you are an artist. Then I don't need to tell you about loss. It's the air you breathe, the bread you eat, which is why you are an artist. If your medium is film, then shoot away.

Grandma told me she named one of the geckos Joyce, and another one Elaine. There are more than two of them, running along the eaves under the tile roof and up the mural of sunset over the Gulf of Papagayo, but just two with names. This week was the first time I ever saw geckos in the flesh. They are as cute as the Geico gecko, but not as big. No way could they reach the gas pedal on his Geico car. They probably run faster than his little car anyway.

There are more dogs than people in Playas del Coco. Patricia and Antonello's dog, Indy (aka Indiana Jones) came to dinner last night. He lives across the street and up the hill now, over-looking the Gulf, but he still gets confused. He stayed in the dining room, in case you are concerned about the sanitation issue. He knows better than to get in the way of the ladies in the kitchen. They move even faster than the geckos and are much bigger. Plus, they carry knives.

The most entertaining of the animals we watch from the family table are the iguanas, Arturo One, Arturo Two, Arturo Three, and Arturo Four. You'd think there would be a girl in the bunch. But Richie didn't check before he named them.

The hibiscus twigs along the boundary wall come to within eight inches of the tin roof. Right now they do, anyway. Things grow pretty fast around here. The Voodoo Princess says they are halfway through the machete/bald and jungle/overgrown cycle. For now, it's a good three feet (or nearly one meter, since we're in Costa Rica—did I mention that?) to any substantial branch that could support an adult iguana.

Yesterday, I was sitting at the family table sipping an Imperial, the national beer, scribbling maniacally on a yellow legal pad about gallbladders, when I heard this scrambling noise of nails on tin overhead, and then, suddenly, silence, except for the shaking of the hibiscus. I looked up and scanned the hedge to find one of the Arturos, who had leapt from said tin roof to said hibiscus and was celebrating by eating a hibiscus flower. It looked quite tasty, the color of watermelon.

However, that's not the only way the leap could go. Life is full of many possibilities beyond our poor plans or even our poor imaginations. You can be born in a little town in Oklahoma, get blown out of there by drought and depression, driven by the great economic engine to all parts of the twentieth century, and end up in the twenty-first in Costa Rica.

This morning after my walk with Dr. Will, I was again sitting at the family table with a cup of coffee and my legal pad. I heard the scrambling noise, jerked my head up to the hibiscus hedge. But—no shaking. The silence was interrupted. *Plop*. Ah, Richie told me what that sound meant—a different possibility. I looked down. Sure enough, there was an Arturo on the ground. He barely missed the tile. Shall we pause to give thanks for one possibility that did not come to pass?—*splat*. Not today. He raised his head. But he stood still. Looked a little winded, actually. A full minute later he turned his head to the left. Yes, that still worked. Then to the right. That worked too. He blinked a few times. "Where am I?" I watched the cloudiness fade from his brow. "Oh, yes, I've been here before." He took another breath, moved one limb, then another, then another, then his tail, then took a few tentative steps.

I expected him to scoot over to the hibiscus hedge. Nope. Evidently, you get a blossom only if you are successful in your leap. He climbed back up the wall to the roof and disappeared.

But he *was* successful. He survived. He can leap again tomorrow.

He *will* leap again tomorrow.

A Voice from the Edge

Jump!

The week after my return from Costa Rica I had another doctor's appointment, this one with my regular doctor, and I said not a word about bizarre thoughts or nail files. I got a new script and was off on my next adventure, this one called Celexa.

I did the laundry and packed my new meds for a business trip. For the life of me, I cannot tell you where I went, some conference, some hotel . . . Cincinnati? I do remember the balconies on each floor overlooking the lobby. Right outside my room, I leaned over the rail. I don't know why I even had a room. I never slept on Celexa.

The hard marble fountain in the lobby looked lovely from up on the fourteenth floor as I leaned over, gripping the rail. The fountain called me to come down.

But wait. Directly below me was the roof over the fitness center. Sure, it was thirteen flights down. But what if its slope broke my fall? What if the fall didn't kill me? I could end up paralyzed. If paralyzed, how could I carry out my plan?

Besides, ow.

Do antidepressants prevent suicide? Or do they raise the risk?

Yes.

That is why I started taking Prozac, because I was thinking about suicide. I didn't have a plan back in November 2004. I certainly didn't plan to use my plan. But when George was reelected, my doc said St. John's wort and fish oil were clearly not cutting it. It was time to haul in a big gun. Prozac is cheap, and back then people were popping it like M&M's. I don't know, maybe they still are.

Soon I was cranky, distracted, anxious, and I couldn't sit still. As I said, we decided I needed more Prozac. Then I was pushing a nail file into my neck while driving down the highway.

On Celexa, I leaned over guardrails in hotels. On Cymbalta, I stopped eating, hoping I would disappear. I stopped sleeping, stopped caring when my car drifted into the path of eighteen-wheelers. I raged at my shrink. On Effexor, my fingers, well, every cell in my body was shaking. I became convinced I needed to remove the blood from my body, if not in the ER, then in my kitchen, so I could get the drug out of my blood, since obviously my psychiatrist was poisoning me. For two years I "kept trying" antidepressants and only felt better each time when I stopped.

Each and every one of these near misses occurred during a classic "mixed episode," a combination of manic and depressive symptoms. Sixty-three percent of the people who attempt suicide do so while experiencing either a mixed episode of bipolar or what they call "mixed features" in major depression.[1]

But in the DSM-IV, there was a condition for these manic symptoms to be considered an indication of bipolar disorder: *The symptoms are* not *due to the direct physiological effects of a substance (e.g., a drug of abuse, a medication, or other treatment) or a general medical condition (e.g., hyperthyroidism).*

I couldn't be diagnosed with bipolar because I was taking antidepressants when I developed its symptoms. The symptoms were considered merely side effects of the medication. So they kept giving me antidepressants, which kept sending me into mixed episodes, because according to the DSM, I still had major depression.

DSM-5 now recognizes bipolar if the full criteria for mania or hypomania are met, even when the symptoms are provoked by an antidepressant, if they persist beyond the antidepressant. In fact, these kinds of reactions, even short of a full-blown mania or hypomania, are taken as clues that the person who experiences them might not have major depression after all, but rather bipolar.

But the DSM-5 wasn't published until 2013.

What if, what if . . .

Whatever.

A Voice from the Edge

Making the Call

We interrupt this program to tell you what on earth we are talking about. About time, you say?

First let's clarify the question.

Do you want to know: *How do I know if I have bipolar?* Or do you want to know: *What the hell is happening to my brain?*

I am guessing you got curious when you or somebody you love ended up with a diagnosis. Is it for real? How did you get the diagnosis, anyway? You had symptoms and subjective experiences and you displayed certain behaviors, that's how. I'll start there. We'll get to the *What the hell is happening* part later.

The *Diagnostic and Statistical Manual* (DSM) is the Big Book of Diagnoses. Big. Really big. Lots of chapters. Bipolar is in the Mood Disorders chapter, along with major depression. There is more to both than mood, as you shall see, but that's where they start.

Bipolar, as you might guess from the name, has two poles, mania/hypomania and depression, the proverbial up and down. Way oversimplified, but it's a start.

Depression is diagnosed from the following signs and symptoms:

At least one of these two:
• Depressed, sad, empty, hopeless mood, or irritable most of the day, nearly every day
• Markedly decreased interest or pleasure in most activities, most part of the day, nearly every day

And then three or four of these:
1. Significant weight loss when not dieting or weight gain
2. Insomnia or oversleeping nearly every day
3. Psychomotor agitation or retardation that others can see
4. Fatigue or loss of energy
5. Feelings of worthlessness or excessive or inappropriate guilt
6. Diminished ability to think or concentrate, or indecisiveness
7. Recurring thoughts of death or suicide, or has a plan, or has attempted suicide

There are some modifiers here: duration, severity, level of impairment. Let somebody else sort it out. They should also rule out effects of substance use or some other medical condition.

This list works like a Chinese menu. The first two, (depressed or irritable mood) *or* (loss of interest or pleasure) are the core symptoms. Next, choose three or four of the remaining seven for a total of five. Notice how often the word *or* appears: weight loss *or* gain, too much *or* not enough sleep, agitation *or* slowing down.

I call depression the Junk Drawer of the DSM. In the world of diagnosis there are lumpers and splitters. The Mood Disorders chapter of the DSM goes to the lumpers. Things that could have been sorted are all lumped together, because . . . well, frankly because the DSM's paradigm isn't particularly sophisticated. It's all about mood, which is up or down, and everything else is a tagalong.

If, in the depths of your misery, you don't remember ever

being up, if the doctor you went to because you are tired of being down doesn't happen to observe up, if nobody in your family ever went to a doctor and got diagnosed with bipolar, and if nobody else you know is in the office with you to report the time you wrote a book in three weeks, then you are diagnosed with some variant of unipolar depression, one of which is major depression. "Unipolar" means only one pole, down. No up.

So, what about up? That is how you get the bipolar diagnosis. If you have previously had an episode of depression, then when a doctor finally notices up, an episode of mania or hypomania (mania-lite, in the world of the DSM), or a friend or family member finally reports that particular brand of crazy, you graduate to a new diagnosis. You skip the depression diagnosis and go straight to bipolar if you are being diagnosed while you are bouncing off hospital walls.

Here are the symptoms of a manic episode:

- A distinct period of abnormally and persistently elevated, expansive, or irritable mood, lasting at least one week for most of the day (or any duration if hospitalization is necessary)
- During the period of mood disturbance and increased energy or activity, three or more of the following symptoms have persisted (four if the mood is only irritable) and have been present to a significant degree and are different from usual behavior:
    1. Inflated self-esteem or grandiosity
    2. Decreased need for sleep (e.g., feels rested after only three hours of sleep)
    3. More talkative than usual or pressure to keep talking
    4. Flight of ideas or subjective experience that thoughts are racing
    5. Distractibility (attention too easily drawn to unimportant or irrelevant external stimuli)

6. Increase in goal-directed activity (socially, at work or school, or sexually) or psychomotor agitation
7. Excessive involvement in pleasurable activities that have a high potential for painful consequences (e.g., unrestrained buying sprees, sexual indiscretions, or foolish business investments)

Did you notice that "psychomotor agitation" and "distract-ibility" from the mania list look an awful lot like "psychomotor agitation" and "diminished ability to concentrate" from the depression list? If you are confused, don't worry. So is the DSM.

The differences between mania and hypomania are length and severity. They use the same set of symptoms to describe hypomania, only the time required for diagnosis is four days, not seven, and the way it manifests does not get you arrested, fired, divorced, hospitalized, or psychotic. The "arrested, fired, divorced, hospitalized, or psychotic" variety is Bipolar I. The merely disturbing is Bipolar II.

When you have a previous episode of depression, followed by a manic or hypomanic episode, they make the call. Again notice that unless your first diagnosis is made in the hospital or by a doc who is looking more carefully than most for other subtle signs (more on these later), or you have a blazing family history of the disorder, you don't get to this diagnosis until first you have been *mis*diagnosed with unipolar depression and given antidepressants that can make you crazy and will eventually worsen the course of the disorder. Isn't this fun.

If you have some of these manic symptoms, but not enough, or not enough days in a row, they are deemed not relevant. If these symptoms come during a depressive episode, they still call it depression but add the qualifier "with mixed features." I said I had "mixed episodes" in the last chapter. It looks the same, but they save "mixed episode" for after they have switched your diagnosis to bipolar. They hadn't recognized my trip to Costa

Rica as hypomanic yet. Many docs believe bipolar is rare, it is scary, you don't want that diagnosis, and they don't want to "overdiagnose" it. Instead, they keep giving you antidepressants until the ironclad case can be made.

Imagine this were cancer. You don't want that diagnosis, either. But oncologists manage to pull up their big girl panties, investigate the possibility, break the news, and get their patients to the appropriate treatment.

Bipolar disorder is not diagnosed and not treated appropriately for an average of 7.5 years,[1] during which patients are test tubes in our own personal chemistry experiments, while doctors keep changing the antidepressants that keep flipping us into mixed episodes and everybody else tells us to keep trying.

Often, the correct diagnosis is made when the patient on antidepressants switches from depression to full-blown mania. Some doctors do pay attention after enough mixed episodes. It helps to see a doc at a center that specializes in bipolar because they are already paying attention. But when the local shrink is perfectly willing to say you are depressed, and depressed sounds pretty normal to you, because isn't everybody these days, why go searching for worse news?

This is why.

Mixed episodes combine the worst of depression with the extra energy of bipolar. You are already in some circle of hell when you get this power surge that pounds you even lower. I mean, it's one thing to be depressed, in your pajamas, stuck to the sofa, stuffing your face with Cheetos, and thinking about nail files or guardrails. Or the gun in the nightstand. It is quite another suddenly to have both the energy and the impulse to jump up and do something about it.

Mood doesn't capture it. It's the energy that will kill you. Pay attention to the energy.

Cymbalta actually sounds the alarm. Well, it raises a finger, in the prescribing sheet.

*The following symptoms, **anxiety, agitation, panic attacks, insomnia, irritability, hostility, aggressiveness, impulsivity, akathisia (psychomotor restlessness), hypomania, and mania,** have been reported in adult and pediatric patients being treated with antidepressants for major depressive disorder as well as for other indications, both psychiatric and nonpsychiatric. Although a causal link between the emergence of such symptoms and either the worsening of depression and/or the emergence of suicidal impulses has not been established, there is concern that such symptoms may represent precursors to emerging suicidality.*

Consideration should be given to changing the therapeutic regimen, including possibly discontinuing the medication, in patients whose depression is persistently worse, or who are experiencing emergent suicidality or symptoms that might be precursors to worsening depression or suicidality, especially if these symptoms are severe, abrupt in onset, or were not part of the patient's presenting symptoms.

Consideration should be given to changing the therapeutic regime . . . Ya think?

Cymbalta is being modest here. Far and away the majority of people who jump over the rail or make some other suicide attempt have these symptoms. Irritability and psychomotor agitation are the strongest predictors of the jump.[2]

The patient information sheets invariably say you should report these symptoms to your doc. I don't know about yours, but mine (my second psychiatrist by the time I was on Cymbalta) told me that **agitation, insomnia, irritation, and psychomotor restlessness** are symptoms of depression, and would go away if I kept taking my meds. So my **hostility** was entirely misplaced.

The real experts in bipolar (Akiskal, Ghaemi, Goodwin, Jamison—there's a bibliography at the back) think the DSM made a mistake back in 1980, when it sorted mood disorders by up/down. The real issue is not up and down but rather cycling. A better way to sort would be between persons who experience one or two episodes of depression and those who experience cycling: up, down, mixed, and stable, in turns. Some, like Phelps and friends (also in the bibliography), say up doesn't have to mean crazy high; it can simply be not as down as usual, which would include those for whom depression goes away and keeps coming back. There are a lot of people in the unipolar depression junk drawer who belong in the bipolar-*ish* drawer. Half the people in the unipolar drawer eventually get switched to the bipolar drawer, anyway.[3] If they live long enough. Researchers estimate that between 25 and 60 percent of persons with either Bipolar I or II attempt suicide at some time in their lives.[4] Those who have access to guns usually die.

This is called the bipolar spectrum,[5] and you won't find it in the DSM. The chair of the DSM-5 effort, David Kupfer, knew about it, wrote about it back in 2003, wanted to include a way to recognize it in this book published in 2013 that will guide diagnosis for the foreseeable future. But enough of the psychiatric community thought it was too complicated that he was overruled.

But your doctor's task is not about avoiding the bipolar diagnosis until denial becomes impossible. It's about getting the right treatment in time to prevent something terrible, or simply to give you your life back before it is disrupted beyond repair. And for those of us on the bipolar spectrum, antidepressants are not the right treatment.

Antidepressants can make us crazy. Have I said it enough?

OK, it is true, some people who have been diagnosed with bipolar do take antidepressants. If that is all they take, they are playing with fire. The standard medications for bipolar are mood stabilizers. Lithium has the strongest record of success, though it works best for those who have the most classic version of

Bipolar I.[6] Its success rate goes down for mixed episodes and the kinds of bipolar that are more frequently misdiagnosed as major depression.[7] There are other choices as well. Everybody is different, right? The docs who know what they are doing first prescribe a mood stabilizer for bipolar. Some augment with an antidepressant, as long as a mood stabilizer is on board. Sometimes the antidepressant seems to help. Not much more than placebo, but sometimes. The experts call this antidepressant-plus-mood-stabilizer approach controversial.[8] Some are willing to try it if they and the patient are desperate.

It continues to amaze me that the pharmaceutical companies do not get on the bipolar spectrum bandwagon and sort this out.[9] In drug trials antidepressants barely beat placebos, and the companies have to fight these continual legal battles over whether their drugs caused the next sorry soul's suicide. If the only people who took antidepressants were those with true unipolar depression who need the chemical kick in the butt, then success rates would rise. That's what antidepressants do, more or less, give you a chemical kick in the butt, or rather, brain. If doctors didn't prescribe antidepressants to people who, you could predict, were going to have bad results once they got the energy surge, the companies wouldn't get sued for those bad results.[10, 11]

And we wouldn't end up pushing sharp objects at our necks.

Of course, all the mood stabilizers, the right medication for bipolar and bipolar-*ish*, have been around for decades and are available as generics, in other words, cheap, while each new antidepressant is a license to print money.

But I am sure the money has nothing to do with it.

Now, I am not a doctor, and I do not know you. Don't take my word for it. But if antidepressants consistently make you crazy, talk to your doctor about the bipolar spectrum. If your doc dismisses your concerns, talk to another doc.

We now return you to our regular programming. Back to Costa Rica, 2005.

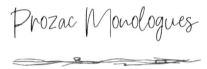

The Fourth Step: In which I turn around

Friday, January 28, 2005

I used to work for a residential treatment center for behaviorally disturbed adolescents. As though we have to remind ourselves that there are no bad children, only children who behave badly. The kids weren't fooled by the euphemisms. They called it "one stop short of juvie jail."

In reality, there are no bad children. But some children are born to severely whacked-out parents, and these children develop a variety of behaviors to accommodate that fact, some of which society does not appreciate and chooses to modify behaviorally.

One of the kids had been locked in the basement of his "home," meaning the place where his whacked-out mother and stepfather resided, for years. They let him out for beatings. The county didn't listen to him whenever he managed to run away and kept sending him back to his parents. In one final escape he committed armed robbery. They didn't hear that as a cry for help either, but it did get him out of the basement. Who is the crazy one here? He turned out to be a compassionate young man, always looked out for the younger kids, encouraged their efforts. He didn't need his behavior modified. The county that sent him back to his parents did.

I am sitting at the newly installed bar at the Pato Loco, listening to Crosby, Stills & Nash in the background, "Helplessly hoping . . ." A dip in the serotonin level here. The Prozac is fading. Or maybe it's the 11 a.m. beer. Am I blue because I drank the beer, or did I drink the beer because I am blue? Frankly, I am blue all the time, but Stephen Stills tends to remind me.

Some kids worked a twelve-step program at this treatment center. But everybody did the center's program. It had seven steps.

Here is how it worked. Every day each kid sat down with a counselor to go over the step he or she was working on. The step was a behavior to be practiced every day for a week. Like leaping from a tin roof to a hibiscus hedge. There was a reward for successful completion. Like eating a hibiscus flower. Not that exactly. They needed rewards even in Iowa winter, and hibiscus doesn't bloom in Iowa winter. But something like it. At the successful completion of the behavior every day for a week, there was a bigger reward in the form of more privileges. Plus, they went on to the next step. This is called positive reinforcement, which in the long run works better than punishment to produce behavior that society appreciates.

The first step was "Ask a question."

Does that sound ludicrously easy? Who can't ask a question? In fact, it is terrifying for somebody who grew up in a house where the only time you are safe is when they forget you are there. In that kind of house, learning to keep your mouth shut is the rewarded behavior. It is explicitly taught, usually with punishment. "Why can't you learn to keep your @#$&%!! mouth shut?" Whack!

But asking a question is a basic life skill for navigating territory you don't know as well as you know your own whacked-out family of origin. If you have trouble asking for directions, you could use this program to get better at this life skill. It helps to ask for directions when you travel. In Playas del Coco, you will find it useful to get yourself to say even to a stranger, "*¿Donde está el servicio, por favor?*" (Where is the bathroom, please?), especially after an afternoon of "*Dos cervezas, por favor*" (Two beers, please).

You might like to practice this asking of questions in a comfortable environment before you try it out in the world. This is what you do. First, break it down:

1. Decide on some information you want.
2. Figure out who has the information.
3. Among those who have the information, choose which person you want to ask.
4. Form the question in words. Include the word "please."
5. Pick a quiet time when that person is not busy.
6. Ask the question. Include the word "please."
7. Listen to the answer.
8. Say "thank you."

Do this every day for a week, and a second week if you don't succeed the first. Or even a third if you need the practice. Be sure to reward yourself after #8. If you have been sucking down cervezas in the hot sun all afternoon, then the location of *el servicio* will be reward enough. If you are going to need paper, you might bring some with you, just in case.

Travel tip: if you go to El Bohio in Playas del Coco, you need to bring your own toilet seat, as well as paper. On the upside, their fried chicken is the cheapest in town. Not the best, mind you, but the cheapest. It is served in front of a fabulous mural painted by the Voodoo Princess and her friend Ceci, who owns El Bohio. The Voodoo Princess needs regular outlets for her creative streak or she gets cranky. Mama's intent, when she bought the Pato Loco, was to feed the world. The Voodoo Princess is using it as a strategy to escape her previous job managing a magnesium processing plant in order to create installation art.

If you go to Bohio for lunch, you will run into Richie taking his midday break, sucking down his dos cervezas, and waiting for the little girl who comes to the table every day to sell him green mangoes with salt. I asked Richie if he likes green mangoes with salt. He said no, but she can't go home until she sells the mangoes.

People come around Bohio selling jewelry of varying quality, bootleg CDs, and amazing indigenous pottery. You hear the latest gringo gossip and watch the whole town come and go across the street at the plaza and post office and police station. Eat at Bohio. Ask your question somewhere else—where they have a toilet seat.

Most kids at the home spent a while on the first step, before they figured out it was a safe place to ask a question and got the hang of the process. I don't remember all seven steps. But the fourth was an arrow to my heart. It was the hardest in the program and the turning point. Once you did the fourth step, you got major new privileges. Like, you could go from building to building unescorted.

This was the program's fourth step: "Ask for help."

Now, I work with a lot of people who have trouble with this particular life skill. They are lucky they never got into enough trouble to get sent to a residential treatment center for behaviorally disturbed adolescents, or they would still be there.

Or maybe they are not lucky. If they had been smart enough to commit armed robbery, they could have gotten help with this skill while young enough to learn new behaviors. I myself was never smart enough to commit armed robbery. Well now, it's not that armed robbery is smart in and of itself, but it was a successful strategy for that abused boy to get to a safer place, which, given his life to that point and the foreseeable future, happened to be jail.

I was never locked in a basement and let out for beatings as a child. So my need was not quite as desperate. Nevertheless, I, too, have difficulty with asking for help. I can ask about the bathroom easily enough. That's the first step. But I once lost fifteen pounds because the cooks at seminary were on strike, and I had to eat in restaurants, but I couldn't bring myself to ask a waiter to serve me. It was bizarre, walking into restaurants hungry and walking out again scared. Oh well. I didn't need those fifteen pounds. Plus, the panic attacks induced by my unsuccessful attempts to order food got me into therapy.

Here is another example of armed robbery as a way to ask for help:

In April 2004, around three o'clock on a Tuesday afternoon, a man walked into a bank in Keokuk, Iowa, a town of about eleven thousand people in the most southeast corner that sticks out from the rest of Iowa like Florida sticks out from the United States. He proceeded to shoot a large caliber handgun into the air and did your basic demand for cash. Then he left, got into his pickup truck, and drove with his newly acquired cash and his large caliber handgun to the police station.

Leaving the cash and the gun in the cab, he walked into the police station and told them he had just robbed a bank. Well, now he had somebody's attention.

He told them he couldn't take it anymore. He didn't need the money. He didn't want the money. He didn't want to hurt anybody, either. What he wanted was to be put in a cell. He said, "The only thing I can live in is an eight-by-eight cell." They put him in one, in the Lee County Jail.

He got what he expected as a consequence of his bank robbery. He had planned and executed this action with great precision to achieve precisely this result.

This gentleman—that's what his friends called him, and even the owner of the bank after he got to know him—was a soldier, thirty-eight years old, from Fort Campbell, Kentucky, a master sergeant in the US Army's 101st Airborne Division. He had left Kentucky eight hours earlier that Tuesday morning. When the army contacted his wife, she was already looking for him. I guess she knew.

I call him a gentleman too, because I agree with everybody else. He thought through the consequences of his actions for both himself and others. He knew he was going to fire shots in the air. He looked for a small-town bank with only one story so nobody on a second floor would get hurt accidentally if bullets went through the ceiling. When he entered the police station, he left his weapon in the truck. That way, the police would not draw theirs when he entered the station, and his training would not kick in. He would not return fire. One more thing, the handgun he used was not issued by the army. It was his own. I'm not sure what his thinking was there. The news account didn't explain.

This soldier had recently returned from Iraq. Maybe you remember stories about the 101st Airborne? Maybe they didn't touch you quite as personally as they did those of us who live in parts of the United States where many young men and women look to the army for a sense of purpose and a future. Whether or not it was what they got out of the deal, twenty thousand soldiers from the 101st shipped out to Kuwait in February 2003. They crossed into Iraq in March 2003. They were in it from the start and served in Iraq for a year. Their job, according to public affairs officer Lt. Col. Trey Cate, was "to provide a secure environment to facilitate the rebuilding of the central government services." That means they went where the environment wasn't already secure.

The 101st Airborne lost fifty-eight men in 2003.

I wonder how many men the 101st lost the way it lost the man who robbed the Keokuk Savings Bank. He was a casualty too. Is anybody keeping count?

I couldn't find out what happened to him. I wonder if he is still in jail, or if he is in therapy. Either way, these are more secure environments than he'd experienced in Iraq, and more secure than he felt even after he got back to Fort Campbell. It was something of a roundabout way, but he asked for help and he got it.

Then there were those young men who tried to rob the bank at Rockaway Beach, Oregon. Was that a cry for help? Were they trying to get out of the house? Or into therapy? If what they wanted was to get some money, then robbing the bank was not smart at all. It was stupid. It was one of those, "Hey! You! Out of the gene pool!" moments.

In late July 2001, the agenda for my family's reunion did not include witnessing a bank robbery. But you never know how things will go. Five brothers and sisters and spouses and children had gathered on the Oregon coast, plus my mother and great aunt Vi. Aunt Vi is fireworks in a wheelchair, unlike Grandma, who is more like pudding. Aunt Vi'll ram you if she thinks you are moving too slow. Brother Kirk was not with us because his champion stallion Catchmeinyourdreams was running a race, earning his way to Santa Anita. Yes, I have a sister who owns a restaurant in Costa Rica and a brother who breeds racehorses in Texas, using surrogate mares and in vitro fertilization. I am not making these people up and haven't even mentioned sister Karla who sells sheep guts. No, there, I have. And a wheelchair-bound aunt who thinks she drives demolition derby. No, the depressive lesbian priest is not the outlier in this family.

Rockaway is on the Pacific Ocean, just like Coco, though it takes a tougher bird to live on the Oregon coast than on the Gulf of Papagayo. There is one road in and out. It runs north and it runs south. One block west, you are in the Pacific Ocean. Three blocks east, you are in brush so thick you can move ten feet an hour if you have a machete and know how to use it. The brush goes on for thirty miles.

On the day in question, the family scattered across six different locations, up and down this one road that runs north and runs south. My nephew Travis and his wife, Christine, were sitting in the fishermen's bar across from the bank, which was open at 9:45 in the morning, the bar, that is, not the bank, this being a resort town. They were later questioned by the authorities, which is not something you can count on for entertainment during your average summer vacation.

Events began earlier that morning, fifteen miles south in one of a series of small towns along this one road, when two young men stopped at a garage across the road from a coffee-roasting establishment operated by the local forest ranger. I don't know what her forest ranger duties entail, but they leave her time to make cappuccinos. She told Helen and me this portion of the story the next day while steaming our milk. The stories run north and run south, like the road, and bind together all these small towns on the Oregon coast.

The young men were driving a red Camaro. They wanted a tune-up. The mechanic did not have time to give them a tune-up. Other people already had morning appointments. But he could do an oil change right then, which they asked him to do.

And that is how it happened that the bank robbers, for that is what they were, or rather intended to be, arrived at the US Bank in Rockaway Beach, Oregon, in their red Camaro at 9:45 a.m. on July 30, 2001. Maybe they planned to get there at 10:00. But they failed to adjust their schedule to compensate for the shorter service time at the garage. They should have stopped across the road from the garage for a cappuccino. Or even a beer in Rockaway. The bar across from the bank was, as I said, already open.

The bank did not open until 10:00. But at 9:45 these eager young men pulled their black ski masks over their faces. Did I mention this was July? When they discovered the door was locked, they knocked.

Now I don't know that the tellers would have opened the bank door for anybody a full fifteen minutes before bank hours.

My guess is they would not be able to record a transaction of any sort before 10 a.m., let alone one as large as the one I would hope these young men had in mind, given the consequences of their actions. But as it happens, the doors were glass. The tellers were particularly disinclined to open the door to two young men whom they could see were wearing black ski masks in July and waving their semiautomatic weapons. Instead, the tellers called the police.

I swear to you, Travis and Christine saw the robbers waving their guns and the tellers shaking their heads.

When the would-be bank robbers heard the alarm and then the sirens, they decided to try again at a later time, which would have made more sense if they had thought of it earlier. They jumped into their red Camaro, the one that needed a tune-up, and headed north toward a series of small towns just like Rockaway, with ocean to the west and brush to the east and sheriff's deputies in every single one. With radios. And usually not much opportunity to use the radios. But they had opportunity that day.

Soon these two young men in their red Camaro had a lot of company. From all directions. There being two.

Because they were not in enough trouble already, they shot at one of the deputies' cars. They did not hit anybody, but flying glass cut one of the officers on the face. Charges were mounting.

The would-be bank robbers found a new subdivision in Wheeler where they could turn east. They traveled at a high rate of speed until they reached the end of the cleared brush, which was three blocks. As I said. At that point, they disappeared into the vegetation.

However, they did not have a machete, and the sheriff's deputies had dogs. It took a while for the dogs to arrive, as well as the helicopter, which also did not usually get a lot of use. This was a big day for law enforcement. But the robbers were no longer traveling at a high rate of speed, as they had no machete. They couldn't have traveled at a high rate of speed even with a machete. But who knows if they might have been a danger to themselves or others if they had thought this caper through to the point that they were going to need a machete. I suppose it is just as well that they did not.

They were prepared with a cell phone. It came in handy to call the sheriff from the top of a tree surrounded by dogs, so they could ask for help.

See, because I think my bizarre thoughts through to their logical conclusions, I myself have never committed armed robbery. In fact, I think my bizarre thoughts through to their logical conclusions so thoroughly that all my various plans, as in "Do you have a 'plan'?" are carefully designed to minimize the trauma inflicted on law enforcement. Maybe that's why I feel connected to the master sergeant who left his gun in the truck. I have to get my help by asking for it.

And I did. I spent all last week asking for help every single day.

Monday, I made the appointment and saw the second doctor. I found out the reason I felt like I was coming down with the flu, my head was spinning, and my skin was crawling was that I had gone off Prozac cold turkey. She recommended Benadryl.

Tuesday, I asked somebody else to do my work at a meeting. When I told her I had become a noncompliant patient and refused to take my Prozac, she said, "Being noncompliant is the precious option of a thinking woman." I need that woman for my sensei. Then I took the Benadryl, slept, and watched *Seinfeld* reruns all day.

Wednesday, I skipped a class that I teach. But I am extremely responsible and always make sure all my responsibilities are covered. I can't check into the psych ward until I do, which has kept me out of the psych ward at least four times, including the day when I did not stab my doctor so I could attend the Annual Meeting.

Thursday, I made an appointment with my real doctor for when I get back from Costa Rica. I will tell her about my bizarre thoughts, though I will leave out the details of interest to her personally. I don't want to cloud her judgment.

Friday, I finally called a therapist. She's not a new therapist. She is somebody I have seen before with Helen and my son, Jacob, when I wasn't feeling so bad but they were, at least with each other. Helen says it would have been easier to stepparent if she had met Jacob earlier when he was toddler-cute, instead of on the brink of adolescence. I won't have to start from the beginning with this therapist. I have had depression before, plus a divorce, which was very depressing, though not near as depressing as the marriage. I have told my story a lot to therapists and lawyers and judges, and I am tired of it, because depression really is very boring. When we talked on the phone, the therapist sounded glad to hear from me again, and said this (therapy) was going to be good. That cheered me up a lot. Besides being tired of my story, I am also tired of people who feel sad for me when I tell it.

Saturday an old friend asked how I was, and I told him the truth. Since I am having a hard time praying lately, he volunteered to say my prayers for me.

That is six days in a row asking for help. The program says to practice the behavior every day for a week, and I am one day short. But then it was Sunday, and I keep Sabbath. So I packed my bag to receive my reward and flew to Costa Rica.

What a great program! You should try it.

It might be a while before I can handle knives without supervision. But I think when we get back, Helen will allow me out of the house unescorted.

A Voice from the Edge

Three

Have you noticed a theme here? *Increase in goal-directed activity, flight of ideas, distractibility, talking fast/pressure to keep talking, decreased need for sleep*—they are all symptoms of a serious mental disorder and also kind of . . . fun. Yellow notepad, sofa, reality TV, air fresheners, shih tzu, SUV, inspirational posters, air pollution, taxes, 9/11, German tourists, pork chops, laundry, leaping lizards, hibiscus flowers, bank robbery, another bank robbery, another bank robbery . . . Well, I had fun.

The thing about hypomania, when it's good, when it shows up as *elevated or expansive mood* (not irritable) and *increase in goal-directed activity*, as in, *can't stop working on that project*, it is very good. It can turn you into the life of the party and the boss's favorite employee.

Nobody goes to the doc to complain, "They fell out of their chairs laughing at my bank robbery story," or, "I wrote a book in three weeks."

No, we go to the doc in our deepest darkest. At that point, given the memory impairments of depression,[1] the question "Have you ever been manic?" is simply silly. "Have you ever been hypomanic?" is even sillier. In one study that reappraised previous diagnoses, only 22 percent of those with a previous manic or hypomanic episode even recognized it.[2] Nobody asked *me* if I had ever been hypomanic. I wouldn't have known what they meant.

No, I was excited.

Defending themselves from responsibility for seven or more years of suffering and deterioration caused by misdiagnosis and mistreatment, doctors say Bipolar II is tough to diagnose. When you have a condition with different symptoms that come and go in cycles, it's a crapshoot whether it's up or down that shows up on any given day in the doctor's office. And the dice are loaded against the up option, on account of "Nobody goes to the doc to complain . . ." Yes, we have heard it before. For that matter, people with Bipolar II spend more time in depression than in hypomania. Forty times more time. Forty times. With those odds, how are docs supposed to distinguish between somebody who has plain old vanilla depression and somebody who can't remember ever feeling better than the bottom of a sticky shoe but might really have bipolar after all? Like, before you take antidepressants and get worse for seven years until the police escort you to the hospital and somebody finally figures it out.

The docs who know bipolar have found ways around the loaded dice.

A couple years after my trip to Costa Rica, I sat next to a family physician in an airplane. He was curious about the *American Journal of Psychiatry* in my lap. I told him about *Prozac Monologues* and my continued research into what I still thought was my major depression. Whether it was the story itself, or the way I told it, or maybe the volume at which I recounted my medical history to a total stranger on an airplane, he suggested I google "MDQ" when I got home. Which I did.

MDQ turned out to be the Mood Disorder Questionnaire, and I didn't like the results it gave me, different from the plain old vanilla major depression diagnosis three psychiatrists had already made. So, I didn't mention it to my therapist or my doc, which they tell you to at the bottom of the questionnaire, until I was on my fourth psychiatrist and past desperate. But it shaved a few years off that average of seven years' misdiagnosis once I did. The MDQ is used around the world to screen for bipolar and takes five minutes to fill out, so it baffles me why family physicians and even psychiatrists don't use it before prescribing the next pricey new antidepressant.

I am sure the money has nothing to do with it.

There's a copy of the MDQ at the back of this book. Fill it out for yourself. Then have the family member or friend closest to you fill it out, as well, describing his/her observations of you. Sometimes behavior you think is "exciting," like writing a book in three weeks, other people find "disturbing." That's why the MDQ wants to know what other people think too.

Nassir Ghaemi and Ronald Pies, both professors in psychiatry at Tufts University, use a story. It starts, "Some individuals notice that their mood and/or energy levels shift drastically from time to time___. These individuals notice that, at times, their mood and/or energy level is very low, and at other times, very high___." It continues to describe these hypothetical individuals. You check the sentences that sound like you and then score points for how well they describe you. Add up the points. Your score tells you how likely it is you really do need to check this out further.[3]

That's the Bipolar Spectrum Disorder Scale, BSDS. It's at the back of this book too.

Hagop Akiskal, professor of psychiatry and director of the International Mood Center at the University of California at San Diego, has his own approach, called "The Rule of Three."[4] The Rule of Three operates on the insight that many aspects of bipolar actually offer some advantage. Now there is a concept worth exploring. People with bipolar, in our love of excess, have rich and varied life histories. Yes, let's put it that way, rich and varied life histories. Google "famous people with bipolar."

Akiskal works off that insight and probes for threes: three changes of profession or religion, excels in three sports or three musical instruments, speaks three languages. The last one works only for the US-born, because what do you call somebody who speaks only one language? An American.

There are other less attractive examples: three divorces, dated three different people on the same day, three unfinished degrees, three failed antidepressants (sigh), three provoked car accidents. Sexual promiscuity falls under the same rubric, but the bar is set way higher than three. Yeah, if you are mentally counting them up, don't worry. Well, come to think of it, I don't know how far you have counted.

You get the idea. The Rule of Three.

The color red is Akiskal's second criterion, as in "red flag." People with bipolar have flamboyant tendencies, which may show up in things like colorful dress or using a red pen to sign your name. I suppose the red pen thing doesn't work for grade school teachers or editors. Context, people, context.

The red flag only applies to people who slump in their chairs at the doctor's office, complaining of depression, not to happy, healthy overachievers. Again, pay attention to context. Red is not a red flag on a clown. A red wedding dress, or the nun's brilliant lipstick, however, is worth investigating.

Hmm. I got my first red shoes as soon as I could walk and threw such a hissy fit when our dog Fritzi chewed them up that Grandma had to go out and replace them the same day. I have three pair of red shoes in my closet, and one on my feet, right this minute. Does that count?

Prozac Monologues

Slack: In which I give myself room to maneuver

Sunday, January 30, 2005

My vacation book for the middle of these sleepless nights has been *The Lord is My Shepherd: Healing Wisdom of the Twenty-third Psalm*, by Harold Kushner (of *When Bad Things Happen to Good People* fame). Chapter 7 is titled "He Guides Me in Straight Paths for His Name's Sake." Kushner writes, "the Hebrew phrase translated 'straight paths' actually says something complex and more interesting than the translation would convey. It literally means 'roundabout ways that end up in the right direction.'" Then Kushner adds his personal commentary, "I can relate to that."

I think I get it. The young man who committed armed robbery to get out of his abusive household was using a "roundabout way that ends up in the right direction." Not that I recommend committing armed robbery as a way to ask for help. Understand me. If you set out on a roundabout way carrying a loaded weapon, you dramatically decrease the possibility you will arrive anywhere at all. Given how many roundabout ways I tend to travel, I think it best I not even own a weapon.

The passage makes me ponder the roundabout ways of my own life. I recognize its wisdom, its *healing* wisdom, and try to apply it to my judgments of others' wayward ways. But I am not always wise about myself. I don't cut myself slack when I go wayward. That's what I call it, "slack."

See, the shortest distance between two points is not necessarily a straight line. Sometimes there's a roadblock between two points, and the shortest distance is around it, and if you refuse to deviate from your straight and narrow line, you get stuck at the roadblock and never get anywhere, except to the roadblock, of course, which doesn't sound particularly interesting to me, and I suspect is not what you had in mind when you started out this morning.

Like, how trying to be perfect made me far from it.

Or sometimes these deviations are simply about having fun. Like when the color purple is out in left field, and God weeps when you fail to notice it, because it was so much fun creating the color purple and God just wants you to enjoy it too.

Like, why can't I do something for no other reason than fun?

One needs to exercise subtlety of mind to determine how much slack is needed in a given situation. Sometimes it is important to limit slack. For example, if a bucking Brahma bull is placed in a chute with a lot of slack, then the bull can kick the chute apart before the cowboy can even mount, much less get released into the rodeo ring, where the bull can buck to beat Moses without doing as much damage, because there is enough slack, in fact no damage at all, if it goes the way the cowboy and clown and bullfighters intend.

I have no idea how they get that Brahma bull into the little chute to begin with. Grandpa was a cowboy. Not the kind who rode bulls but the kind who raised them. This was in Texas, after he and Grandma blew out of Oklahoma in the 1930s. When Jacob was eight and found out Grandpa was a cowboy, he asked how he got a big bull from one pasture to another. Grandpa said, "You put him there before he gets big." That belongs in a book of cowboy wisdom, like "Don't squat with your spurs on."

There's another piece of cowboy wisdom that goes, "Good judgment comes from experience, and a lotta experience comes from bad judgment." Maybe that's why Grandpa quit ranching and became a carpenter. He seemed more in his element with levels and plumb lines. I don't know how many times he asked me if I knew what a plumb line was. It's in the Bible, the prophet Amos. I think he liked Amos because it's about God being angry at people who don't measure up. Carpenter wisdom is, "Measure twice, cut once."

It was hard to measure up around Grandpa.

Which reminds me, when Grandpa, a lay leader in the Methodist Church and lifelong teetotaler, was on his deathbed, he was nervous, scared actually, about what waited for him on the other side. I wonder, what was the bucking Brahma bull in his life that he wished he had transferred to the pasture where he wanted it before it got big?

Pastures are nice roomy places to go looking for the color purple, or bucking, or whatever it is you want or need to do. But as I was saying, you want to give Brahma bulls very little slack in the chute. The soldier who committed armed robbery in Keokuk, Iowa—he needed a narrow chute for a while to heal. Eight-by-eight he thought would be the right size. I don't know whether he had trouble asking for help, or if he had asked already, but because it was the army, he needed to shout.

Now, kites fall if they have any slack at all. It's sad to see, first the wobble and then the headlong plunge. Ironically, for a kite to rise, first you pull it down. That's what the pre-launch running is about, taking away slack. Then you give it a little slack and take it away again, letting out more string each time. Kites are entirely dependent on the one who holds the string. Like how people who cannot promise not to hurt themselves are entirely dependent on the doctor who gives them The Look.

I once knew somebody who loved kites. When she was a little girl and her kite was way up high in the air, because she was exceptionally good at flying them, her father came up behind her and cut the string. Then the kite had too much slack. So it fell. I think her father did it to remind the little girl that he had a string tied to her, a string with no slack. She fell, too, though in a different way. The result was bad for both the little girl and her kite.

See what I mean? Some situations call for more slack, some less.

I have been thinking about slack my whole life as a parent. When Jacob was born, the nurse told me that newborns feel safest with almost no slack. They like to be swaddled. She taught me how to wrap the blanket around him so his arms and legs were held in place, like in the womb. He did seem to like it. It helped him make the transition from one secure environment to another that was less secure, but that he would learn to navigate soon enough.

She said as soon as babies kick the swaddling off, it's time to leave it off. That is the last self-regulating bit of parenting advice you get. Nine months later, I watched him navigate a short flight of stairs. He had barely begun to crawl, and suddenly he was climbing. He was grinning from ear to ear, while I was in high anxiety. What if he fell?

But I had to let him climb. It was his destiny to climb. So, while he worked his way up, laughing out loud for the sheer joy of his accomplishment, I hovered, recalibrating with each step the distance to the floor and the depth of the carpet. "How far can I let him fall?" Twenty years later, I still wonder, "How far can I let him fall?" The specific calibration changes as the child grows. But the principle remains.

When Jacob was six, he and I lived in a small town in the middle of Iowa. It was a safe place for me to exercise my parenting style, which I call "a long leash." That's another way of describing slack. Most everybody for a several-block radius knew who he was and where he was supposed to be and would make sure he got there when he was supposed to arrive. He had recently learned to ride a bike, which, notwithstanding the neighborly neighborhood, brought the "How far can I let him fall?" thing to a whole new level.

On the day in question, I wasn't sure about letting him ride his bike to the park by himself. It was only two blocks away but in the wrong direction, where not everybody knew who he was and where he was supposed to be. It was the first time he would go anywhere on his bike by himself, except for around the block without crossing any streets, which was nerve-wracking enough for me the first time I'd let him do it and not that long ago. I still wasn't used to the notion of him on his bike not in my direct line of sight. Sometimes parents say "No" because the parents aren't ready, not because the children aren't. But really, I wasn't sure either of us was.

Nevertheless, we talked it over, the stuff about not taking off his helmet, not changing his plans, not going anywhere with anybody else. I gave him fifteen minutes. I gave him my watch so he could tell when he was supposed to be back. I moved the hands on the watch so it would be easy to read. I showed him where the hands would point in fifteen minutes. I checked his helmet. And I waved him off.

Then I sat on the front porch swing to wait. That's the kind of town this was—we had a front porch swing. But this was my baby I had sent out into the wide world by himself, armed with only a helmet and a wristwatch. While I waited, I composed two speeches, one for if he came back in fifteen minutes, one for if he didn't.

He didn't.

At twenty minutes I got on my own bike. I rode to the park. I didn't find him. I rode back home and around the corner to his best friend's house. There was Jacob's bike, leaning against the garage. He never even crossed the street.

Then I rode home. That gave me time for a few deep breaths. I called the friend's house and asked for Jacob. When he came to the phone I said, "Get your butt home now." Then I hung up. That gave him something to think about during the trip while I polished the second speech.

When he arrived, we sat on the front porch swing and I delivered the second speech. "I made a mistake. I thought you were old enough to go the park by yourself and come home when you promised. I was wrong. We will wait until you are older before we try this again." I was proud of my speech. Breathing helped.

Are you following me? I allowed a little slack, like on a kite. But the wind didn't catch it. So I pulled back when the kite wobbled. Give a little slack, let the kite up, pull back when it wobbles. Over the years, that kite has flown higher and higher. We went through a time when we disagreed about who should hold the string. Now he does, but he still asks me to watch. It's a sight to behold.

I'm in Houston now on my way home from Playas del Coco. When my cell phone worked again, I called Jacob. We talked about this story. He said, "I thought it was about safety. But it wasn't. It was about being trustworthy." I told him about Rabbi Kushner's book, and said his detour to his friend's house was a roundabout way that ended up in the right direction. Because today he is exceedingly trustworthy.

My long-leash parenting style is an adjustment to my mother's style. William Strauss wrote a book, *Generations: The History of America's Future, 1584 to 2069*. In it, he attributes the cycles of history, like wars, crime rates, and public investment in education to the same phenomenon, each generation adjusting its parenting style in response to dissatisfaction with the parenting it received. These cycles repeat roughly every eighty years. Strauss claims he can predict future trends, not just explain past ones. He wrote *Generations* in 1991, and things are turning out as one might expect by his theory. This is not good news for the first few decades of the twenty-first century. Remember the 1930s and '40s.

I won't take it personally if Jacob adjusts his parenting style to be different from mine, even if today he says he doesn't need to.

My mother gave her children a lot of slack, you might say "off leash," which wouldn't surprise William Strauss, given her generation. I went to Europe the summer I was nineteen to work in a hotel in Liechtenstein. It was years later before she ever found out I hitchhiked most of the way from London. She had it in her head that I went on some tour. I don't know where she got that idea. I didn't lie. She never asked. Given the parenting I was used to, I didn't notice that she didn't ask. It never occurred to me to tell her.

On the other hand, Mama taught her children by word and example not to cut ourselves slack. This woman learned self-hypnosis to deliver her last two babies, before Lamaze was a thing, and never takes novocaine when she has dental work done because she doesn't want to drool. No slack for *her* spit. At least three of her children have experienced serious health complications on account of our high tolerance for pain. I went to the emergency room once with abdominal pain. When they diagnosed flu, I went home thinking, *This is why people complain so much about the flu.* My appendix ruptured four days later. I felt better then, until three days passed and the abscess that had formed around the rupture was itself about to rupture. The hospital figured it out the next time I appeared at the ER. My mother felt guilty because when we talked on the phone that week, she failed to diagnose appendicitis by the sound of my voice.

Since then, I have lowered my tolerance for pain. I ended up raising a child who has no tolerance for pain whatsoever. I let him stay home from school more days in his twenty years than I have allowed myself to stay home in fifty-two. Following Strauss's theory, I guess I'll start looking now for "Perfect Attendance" pins for my grandchildren.

Cutting myself slack does not come naturally. I wonder if once again I have some abscess around an old wound about to rupture, this time in a psychic sense.

Or back to the kite, I have been pulling harder and harder on my own string until I am no longer up in the air high enough to catch any wind at all.

Mmm. I guess I do need to see a therapist.

It's time to move on.

A Voice from the Edge

Chemistry Experiment

Two days after my return from Costa Rica, it was time for round two, Celexa. But let's skip ahead a year, February 2006, round six.

I'll call my second psychiatrist The Feedbag. She earned a portion of her income from pharmaceutical companies by teaching other psychiatrists about the benefits of their drugs. She was the one conducting round six. She frowned when I called it the Chemistry Experiment.

Then she said, "I get really good results from Effexor."

I said, "What results will *I* get?"

"We won't know until we try it."

Back to the Chemistry Experiment.

Her statement, by the way, is an example of observer bias. The thing about Effexor is, if it works, it is a miracle, and the psychiatrist is a genius. And if it works for you, I truly am glad. If it doesn't, the person taking it quits the psychiatrist who prescribed it. I was one of the latter, at which point this psychiatrist no longer observed me. But she still believed she got great results from Effexor, based on her observation of the patients who told her she was a genius.

I have learned about things like observer bias over the past several years, trying to figure out what the hell happened to my brain. To start, I studied antidepressants, sometimes by reading the research (because even religion majors learn how to do that where I went to college), in addition to my personal Chemistry Experiment.

After Effexor, I put the Chemistry Experiment on hiatus and concentrated on therapy. I still didn't know how far off track I was. And how far off track my doctors were, too.

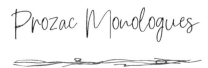

Prozac Monologues

Metaphor: My search for meaning and how the pharmaceutical companies try to help

April 2007

The DSM has its checklists. People with depression have poetry.

People with diabetes discuss their diet, their feet, their retinas. They check glucose levels. Put two diabetics at a table, they compare numbers.

People with depression talk in metaphor. We talk about the cloud, the curtain, the weight, the darkness. When it goes away, we say, "It lifted!" That lift is a physical sensation, actually, of lightness or elevation.

We are drawn to writing, us depressives. Edgar Allan Poe, Virginia Woolf, Sylvia Plath, Ernest Hemingway, Anne Rice—these are writers off the top of my head who had depression or bipolar. People who are depressed want words.

If I could just find the right words, maybe I could break the spell.

The pharmaceutical companies want to help. Truly they do. In addition to the pharmacological options they have for sale, they offer up words to those who are searching for somebody, anybody, who understands our experience.

Do you remember the "Depression hurts" commercials? "The emotional and painful physical symptoms of depression," they said. Not one mental health care professional has ever asked me about pain. It's not one of the diagnostic criteria because the information doesn't help the doctor make the diagnosis; there are so many other things that cause pain. It would, however, tell the patient that the doctor knows what depression feels like. Which would help, actually. Part of the spell is the isolation, the sense that nobody knows, not really. I can't show you an X-ray or a blood test. All I have is words. Do you really believe my words?

It's not like physical pain is the major deal. Until I heard "the painful physical symptoms," I never thought about the pain. It turns out they meant headaches and muscle tension, not the crushing weight on my chest. But before I went to DepressionHurts.com expecting somebody who "got it," I was temporarily lifted from my isolation. The next time I tried to tell somebody, I had new words: "I know my depression is back because my heart hurts."

Ads for antidepressants feature people who feel fabulous. Now they take whatever, and they say "I have my life back." That's a powerful line. But you have to have a neurological receptor for it, some sprig of hope that you, too, can get your life back, once you find the right antidepressant. At times, that proposition seems dubious, and you are at risk for noncompliance, which is when you don't see things the way your doctor does, and you follow your own instinct, which may or may not be the better one.

Then there is the "low incidence of sexual side effects" ad. For that ad to get you to talk to your doctor, you have to want sex enough to admit you're not having any now. It works better on people who are taking something else, already better enough to be bothered by the sexual side effects of their current medication and now willing to pay the hefty co-pay for one that claims not to have them and that their health insurance company isn't crazy about paying for. In which case, good for them.

I nominate "Depression hurts" for a Clio Award (like the Emmys, but for commercials). After the initial grabber, they pile it on, color tones of sepia and gray. (There's a symptom not included in the diagnostic criteria—when the color fades.) "Who does depression hurt?" they ask. "Everybody." The children look at you over their shoulders from the other room, trying not to bother you. The dog holds his leash in his mouth, so patient, so sad. Just like my dog. I didn't walk her today. Again.

So sad. Actually, that's good. Telling the bad news builds trust. Unless I know that you know the bad news and are brave enough to acknowledge it, I don't trust you when you say there's good news. When you try to cheer me up, then I think you haven't a clue. At best you think your cheeriness will help me snap out of it. Snap out of that delusion, yourself. More likely, you're cheering yourself up, because my depression makes *you* feel bad. It's about you. "Depression hurts" is about me.

The other thing about "Depression hurts"—for the first few months the ad ran, it had no name. The product was never, ever mentioned, just the website. Like it's not a commercial; it's a public service announcement.

One day I bit. Cymbalta. Hand it to Eli Lilly. They know marketing.

That's not necessarily bad. It's a complicated strategy, a complicated website, filled with ambiguity. Words about depression are filled with ambiguity.

Not everybody with depression is a writer. Some have hardly any words at all. Healthcare providers have to translate our few and distorted words, or even just our behavior, into the facts of the matter. Children don't say they have "lost interest."

They set their school on fire. Some adults cannot make the word "sad" or "angry" come out of their mouths.

DepressionHurts.com helps.[1] It has this interactive image of a human body. You click on a body part, and up pop questions that you answer on a 0 to 10 scale, questions about sleep, weight, thoughts of hurting yourself, body aches and pains, all the diagnostic criteria, and more. They give you nouns. They let you use numbers; you don't even need adjectives. When you are finished, you review your answers to check if you left anything out. Print the results and take them to your doctor. Then you can nod or shake your head. This is good, even for people who use words. You don't have a lot of energy for words when you have depression. And some of them are hard to say.

I would like the interactive body better if I could pick the gender. Actually, I'm not sure what gender it is. The body is male and the head female? The head freaks me out. It's animated; it grows and turns to face me, then it turns away. Why does it turn away? Does it not like me? I can't determine its ethnicity. It looks like an extraterrestrial.

Maybe they could get software from Lands' End. At the Lands' End website,[2] you create your own virtual model, height, weight, race, skin tone, hair length, wide or narrow hips and thighs, gender. Then you try clothes on your virtual self and rotate to see if the swimsuit makes your butt look fat. You can adjust your numbers to imagine you will lose five pounds between now and when the swimsuit is delivered.

Now why would I mention weight loss to my doctor? At Lands' End, it's an improvement. Again, DepressionHurts.com helps people communicate.

You can even sign up to receive a story every week about somebody who takes Cymbalta. They are nice stories. They are about people like you. They have happy endings.

I tried an experiment. I said I had unexplained headaches at 2 on the scale of 0 to 10, sleeplessness at 2, extra stress lately at

4, and otherwise felt fine. I think I'd feel fabulous if those were my real numbers. When the website added it up, it said I should talk to my doctor about whether Cymbalta would help. Props to Eli Lilly for communication, but let's remember it's a commercial interest operating this website.

Have you tried Cymbalta? How is that experiment working for you?

Do you ever stand in the drugstore, staring at your script, and wonder how that medication and your name came to be connected? Let's step back and trace the history of the Chemistry Experiment, everybody's, that is, not my personal one or yours.[3]

Once upon a time, there was Thorazine. They used it for psychosis, not depression. There wasn't any medication for depressed people unless you count phenobarbital. People with depression either talked it out or snapped out of it. Thorazine is a nasty drug, but it kept psychotic people from committing suicide. It kept them from doing most things they were previously inclined to do, like get out of bed, look at other human beings, lift their feet when they walk. Plus, it turned their skin orange. And made them twitch. Thorazine has so many side effects they list them alphabetically. People didn't take it unless the alternative was suicide.

Nevertheless, the company that sold Thorazine made buckets of money, even with its terrible side effects, because psychosis is even more terrible, and the alternative was lobotomy—the cost/benefit analysis thing. However, not everybody who took Thorazine agreed with their doctor's cost/benefit analysis, and they became noncompliant if somebody wasn't watching. Other pharmaceutical companies figured they could get a share of the market if they could come up with a product with milder side effects.

Enter imipramine. It turns out imipramine didn't work against psychosis. Eventually they found other meds that do, and give people with psychosis their lives back, as long as they keep taking these new meds with a new, different list of terrible side effects.

Ah, side effects. One way to look at it, there are no side effects, just effects. Some effects are those you intend. Others are the little extras that maybe turn out to be bad news, but maybe good. Like, once upon a time you took aspirin for pain. It also thinned your blood. They called the blood thinning thing a side effect. Nowadays that's why people take aspirin, to thin their blood. That side effect is good news, except for people who take aspirin before surgery and have bleeding problems, in which case it is bad news.

Imipramine was a bust for psychosis. But it had an antidepressant side effect, just the ticket for depressed people, psychotic or not, who didn't have time, money, and insurance for analysis and weren't snapping out of it. A market was born.

Maybe you have heard that depression is a chemical imbalance in the brain? It's a bad explanation, but it does explain how they thought imipramine worked.

There are these chemicals called neurotransmitters hanging out in the synapses (spaces) between your neurons (brain cells). Their job is to move messages from one neuron to the next. Once they finish the job, they go inside the neurons, take a break, and wait for the next message. Imipramine targets three neurotransmitters: serotonin, norepinephrine, and dopamine. It "inhibits the reuptake," which is brain-speak for it keeps the chemicals on the job in the synapses, fewer breaks.

People with depression have less of these chemicals in their synapses, the so-called chemical imbalance. After taking impiramine for about a month, some people start to feel better. If a medication makes what neurotransmitters they have work harder, maybe not enough neurotransmitters is why they felt bad in the first place.

Longer work hours! More productivity! Do we have here an American solution to the problem or what?

Imipramine worked. But . . .

Side effects, lots of side effects. Less than Thorazine but enough to leave room for other pharmaceutical companies to keep trying. One particularly troublesome side effect, overdose can be fatal. Give a depressed person a new suicide method. Oops.

Next came MAOIs, monoamine oxidase inhibitors. MAOIs were invented in the 1950s, same as imipramine. These inventors were after tuberculosis. They developed an antibiotic called iproniazid. But there was a problem. Side effect. It made these poor sufferers of tuberculosis so euphoric they neglected basic self-care, like dressing themselves. Naked people, dancing through tuberculosis wards. Disturbing. But somebody who was interested in depression said, "Aha!"

The side effect of interest is that iproniazid inhibits monoamine oxidase. The body uses monoamine oxidase to metabolize (recycle) used-up neurotransmitters, serotonin, et al. An MAOI inhibits this function, leaving more neurotransmitters on the job for longer, postponing their retirement. Again with the American solution.

But there's another side effect—MAOIs interfere with the metabolism of certain drugs and foods containing tyramine. When tyramine levels rise, blood pressure does too. Symptoms include headache, stiff neck, pounding heart, vomiting, collapse.

Oh, and stroke and death. There is a long list of things that kill you if you eat them while on MAOIs, like wine, beer, and aged scotch or whiskey, which is no surprise, they never want you to take alcohol when you're depressed anyway, but also stuff like soy sauce, tofu, cheese, raisins, sauerkraut, salami, herring, ripe bananas. Chicken left out too long somewhere along the line, maybe before you bought it. You never know if there might be a problem until your head is exploding. Medications like cough syrup and cold remedies. I don't know any depressed person with the energy to keep track of this stuff.

The doc who gave me Effexor suggested an MAOI when Effexor was a bust. I took her suggestion as evidence she really didn't like me. I mean, my favorite pizza place was right across the street from her office, sausage, parmesan, beer . . . stroke. I did consider it as a backup plan, as in, "Yes, I have a plan . . ."

In 1989, Eli Lilly struck pay dirt. They figured out how to inhibit serotonin reuptake while leaving norepinephrine and dopamine alone, which vastly reduced the side effects, on account of those two evidently are crankier when forced to work overtime. Prozac was the first selective serotonin reuptake inhibitor (SSRI), and my experience notwithstanding, for vast numbers it has lifted the cloud. It's not perfect and does still bother people, though usually within tolerable limits. The competition in antidepressant development and sales continues to be about side effects. Because I am not the only person who refuses to take something that makes me feel worse.

But it's not only side effects. It's also about whether it works. Prozac poops out. Yes, it's the technical term, Prozac Poop Out. Along came SNRIs to add back the norepinephrine part of the equation, like Cymbalta and Effexor.

Then there are some miscellaneous ones. Wellbutrin affects norepinephrine and dopamine but not serotonin. Remeron does something else . . .

Now we've got two dozen options, more abbreviations than you can shake a stick at, more under development as I write, and no doubt more for sale as you read. How do our doctors decide which ones we get to try next?

They tell us they take into consideration our specific symptoms, like do we need to be pepped up or calmed down, toxicity and risk of suicide, our age and gender, and their clinical experience, but, well, you kind of wonder. I wonder, anyway. I am on hiatus from the Chemistry Experiment right now. Things started to feel random once we got to round seven and were prescribing a suicide method to a suicidal patient. Well, there was always the hope I would feel better again when I quit . . .

Part of any medication's effect comes from your hope for the effect. Hope improves the odds. It used to be, the doctor's word gave you hope. You had a relationship with the doctor and trusted his or her judgment. Now your health care is your own responsibility, even when you're too depressed to care. The doctor doesn't say, "Take my word for it." It's the pharmaceutical companies who do that.

Not in those words. They use other, more wonderful words, more ambiguous (otherwise they wouldn't be legal) words. They weave spells with their words, and we fall under them, hoping these spells will work.

Welcome to my tour of spell-casting words.

The first antidepressant I took back in 1985 was called Elavil. Doesn't that sound cheerful? It elevated my mood. They don't prescribe Elavil much anymore. Side effects. I didn't know about side effects back then, which might have helped me not be bothered by them. Information is a double-edged sword. It can save your life or it can break the spell. Anyway, as a name, Elavil was not a shabby start.

Prozac stumps me. Maybe because they thought it worked well enough, they didn't need much from the marketing department. It sold itself, even with the prosaic name. Since its introduction, it has come to define the category. Prozac means antidepressant, like Kleenex means paper handkerchief. Come to think of it, Prozac sounds like Kleenex. Maybe that was the plan all along.

Celexa sounds heaven-sent, don't you think? I'm thinking blue skies, drifting clouds, gentle breezes. Guardian angels holding me back from the edge. Or pushing me toward it, as it turned out.

Paxil is a bust, name-wise. I don't know many people who take it. Was it trying to compete with Prozac and overreached?

Zoloft inspired my foray into metaphor. One day I found a CD at home, with the words "Zoloft (sertraline HCl)" on it, a mountain scene on the cover, the requisite blue sky, drifting clouds, sunlight on the mountain peaks, all reflected in a deep lake surrounded by dark trees. Heights, depths, light and shadow, and the name—Zoloft. It makes me think of parasailing.

I thought, "Helen has found this promotional material at the psychiatry research center where she works and brought it home for me to learn about my options." Nope. It was music, Vivaldi's *Four Seasons*, packaged by Pfizer. The back listed "Zoloft's Four Indications":

♫ Major depression
♫ Post-traumatic stress disorder (PTSD)
♫ Panic disorder
♫ Obsessive-compulsive disorder (OCD)

I am not making this up. The bullet points for the four diagnoses for which you might take Zoloft (or rather, prescribe it—the CD was given to doctors) were musical notes. Four Seasons, Four Indications, get it? Which do you suppose is spring?

They are getting better with the words all the time. Cymbalta promises a party and will ease the painful physical side effects, should you sprain your back while doing the limbo.

Enough with these fem names. How about Effexor? Now there is an antidepressant on steroids. They give you Effexor when nothing else works. As in, "I'll fix you, my pretty."

Wellbutrin is back to boring. "Well" is an uninspiring aspiration. But Wellbutrin is a special case—"low incidence of sexual side effects." If you can recover from depression and have sex at the same time, who cares what they call it?

You can tell by the names which are advertised in the general media and which are not. Remeron, Parnate, and Aventyl don't work on television. A rose by any other name would smell as sweet, but you couldn't get sixty dollars a dozen for them on Valentine's Day. Effexor would be less effective if it were called Lousital. In which case, aren't we getting our money's worth, for all the advertising?

A friend in AIDS ministry showed me some condoms with the name of an antiviral drug on the packaging, which seemed like good product placement, so to speak. Antiviral drugs don't have metaphoric names. If you have HIV, you get good at medical speak. The very obscurity of those names increases their effectiveness.

We are, after all, spinning a spell that could keep you or me alive, against a disease that kills 15 percent of those who have it. If you tell me taking my meds while facing east and standing on one foot will improve my odds, I'll give it a shot.

When I dream about my depression, it comes to me as a young man who does not like to be called a disease. He doesn't even like "depression." Who would? I call him "Steve." Winston Churchill called his depression his "black dog." But a dog that wants to kill you is not a dog you want to invite into your house.

I listen to Steve in my dreams because I think he has something important to tell me. He employs such desperate measures to get my attention. Part of me worries about taking antidepressants before I get the message, so he has to come back and tell me louder next time. But couldn't he just send an email?

Prozac Monologues

Limp: On top of everything else, my hip hurts

Thursday, February 10, 2005

"What's wrong with your leg?"

I have two jobs these days, one for the congregation of the dread Annual Meeting, the other for the Episcopal bishop of Iowa. Helen and I got back from Costa Rica on Sunday, I whimpered myself to sleep on Monday, and I went to a bishop's staff meeting on Fat Tuesday, soon to be followed by Ash Wednesday, appropriately enough, given my mood. The Prozac is out of my system, and whatever good it did for me, it is doing no longer.

The staff piled into the bishop's car to go eat pancakes at the cathedral when somebody asked the question.

The bishop answered for me from the front seat, "That's what they used to ask Jacob."

My boss is funny that way. Sometimes he comes across as clueless. But don't count on it. Right after you roll your eyes, he pierces straight to the heart of the matter.

I said, "As a matter of fact, I am writing a book. I'm on the chapter called 'Limp,' and it will end with Jacob." My boss wasn't referring to my son. He meant Jacob in the Bible, son of Isaac, grandson of Abraham. This Jacob once wrestled with an angel through the night, until the angel touched his thigh and knocked it out of joint. Jacob survived the fight, but he limped ever after.

I came home from Costa Rica with a limp. My hip hurt, which it has off and on for twelve years. Over the years, various people have used various systems of thought to answer the question my coworker asked, "What's wrong with your leg?" The first time, when it hurt so bad I had to pause and consider my strategy each time I wanted to get in or out of a car, I was making my living by cleaning houses. One of my customers was a physical therapist. Not your typical physical therapist, she uses a system called "Mechanical Link." Mechanical Link is to regular physical therapy as osteopathic is to regular medicine. The word "regular" indicates a certain power position that "regular" medicine holds, like how citizens of the United States call ourselves "Americans." I can't remember how she explained Mechanical Link. But Blue Cross Blue Shield pays for it, so it can't be too bent. Maybe it's like Canada. Except Canada is 10 percent bent, and Mechanical Link is a little more bent than Canada. OK, I know some Canadians who insist they are at least 15 percent bent. (But they aren't.)

This physical therapist and I did not know each other well. We had been testing each other out, each trying to figure out whether the other could tolerate our respective Bent scores. She once left a note that said she hesitated to tell me, in case I thought she was strange, but the house always felt "good" after I cleaned it. I wrote back that it wasn't strange. But I didn't tell her what I was doing to make it feel "good."

One day she was home while I was cleaning. Since I did not have insurance at the time, because I made my living cleaning houses, I hit her up for a free opinion about my hip. She referred me to a chiropractor whom I did not see until later when I did have insurance. And she recommended a book by Caroline Myss, *You Can Heal Yourself.*

A book was more in my price range, especially when she told me it was in the library. Following Myss's recommendation, I started looking at myself in the mirror several times a day to say, "I don't need [blank] to punish me anymore." When I read the phrase, I knew right away whose name belonged in that blank. Do you have a name you would put there?

I had an ongoing conflict with this person in the blank. Myss said my hip hurt because I was stuck and had to get unstuck to move forward. After a few weeks repeating this affirmation several times a day, I figured out something I could let go of to get on with my life, and not stay stuck. My hip did start to feel better. A bit, anyway.

Then one day I was sitting on a couch next to a friend. She knew my hip hurt, but we weren't talking about that. When I got up, she asked, "How's your hip?" I checked. The pain was gone. I could feel its shadow, where it used to be, but it was gone, and it didn't come back. I asked, "What did you do?" She didn't have words to explain it, so I can't tell you. She could just do it. Nevertheless, she healed my hip.

Do I believe these systems of thought? Who am I to quibble?

The pain came back a couple years later. I had insurance this time and could pay for an orthopedic guy who poked my hip with his finger, and it hurt like heck at one particular spot. He said this was excellent news and was quite pleased with himself to make my hip feel like it had been stuck with a hot poker. That meant I had bursitis. I could get one shot of cortisone or I could do several weeks of physical therapy.

Instant gratification or several weeks of daily self-care? Well hey, I am an American. The choice was obvious. I confess that my faith in his system of thought wavered when he said doctors in his clinic gave each other cortisone shots all the time. But what the heck, shoot me up. He gave me the therapy referral as well, just in case.

The shot took away my pain. It was a miracle. For thirty-six hours.

That's when I learned about physical therapy. As it turned out, my decreasing levels of pain were excellent motivation to keep doing the exercises. I also had ultrasound treatments three times a week. The ultrasound thingy was a metal disk inside a plastic wand wired to a console with a bunch of dials. It sent heat into the hip joint to chase away the inflammation when the technician rubbed it over my hip on top of a lubricating gel. All I felt was a slightly alarming tingle. She said it was difficult for the rays to reach all the way into the joint, which is why it had to be done three times a week.

The console and the dials and the gel and especially the tingle made me think of gadgets sold in the back of comic books. The only time I seriously believed it did anything at all was once when the technician got distracted, left the thing in one spot too long, and it burned me.

After we talked about the weather and tomatoes (the staples of summer small talk in Iowa) about twelve times, I hit a plateau and decided the stress of coming in to the office three times a week to make small talk with a technician while she rubbed my hip with the ultrasound gizmo, which is one of the few things I was not sure I believed in, was increasing the pain in my hip. I decided to discontinue with the gizmo, which had a twenty-five-dollar co-pay anyhow, and do my exercises at home.

Then I found another book by a doctor who had a bad back. This book said you should work with all your systems, except for the surgery one. He explained why surgery made bad backs worse.

I do think everything is connected, and everything works. Though nothing has worked entirely. I made the dietary changes he suggested and added some of his exercises to my repertoire. But I didn't go to India to lie on a big hot rock outside a Buddhist monastery for a year, which is what he did to heal his back, because I was still cleaning houses and didn't have access to the system he participated in that afforded him the airfare and the year off. Plus, he must not have been single-parenting a child in grade school. Unless somebody else took care of the kid for him. Actually, I did participate in the system that afforded him to lie on a hot rock in India for a year. But my part in the system was to do things for him or for people like him, and regularly hand over my twenty-five-dollar co-pays.

As I said, nothing worked entirely. Once in a while what I called my "bursitis" would flare. It helps to have a word when people ask, "What's wrong with your leg?" and a regular medical diagnosis is the one most acceptable in most company. It might make them twitchy if I called it "Fred." This was back when I cared about such things, which obviously I don't anymore. What with all my appointments, I don't have the time. It flared again when I stopped cleaning houses in 2003 and instead worked full-time in jobs that I did while sitting. One of these jobs gave me better health insurance, and I went to the chiropractor, and also the Mechanical Link therapist, which helped a lot and improved my posture, the chiropractor and the therapy, not the sitting. But it did not eliminate the pain. When I told my physical therapist that my goal was to keep the pain under control, she said if my goal was not to be pain-free, I never would be.

Well, OK. But I was raised in a working-class family. And that is a different system of thought. People who have other people clean their houses for them pursue medical care in order to maintain their lifestyle. People who do the housecleaning pursue medical care so they can go to work. Just because I changed my job didn't mean I had changed my thinking. The balance had shifted from going to physical therapy so I could go to work to going to work so I could pay my co-pays. If I were pain-free, she might be pleased with herself. But I might be broke.

A year ago, I did a liver-cleansing diet. I started paying attention to information about food when I was on this diet, and I read somewhere that vegetables in the nightshade family cause inflammation. That's what bursitis is, inflammation in the joint, in this case the hip. I decided after the fasting part of the diet, when I was adding foods back one at a time to find out if I had any food allergies I didn't know about (I don't), that I would continue to not eat tomatoes and potatoes for three months, which was the time it was supposed to take to reduce the inflammation.

I picked up a book once that listed things to do to enhance the quality of your life. Not big things like get a job with health insurance or move to Iowa, but little things like "Only eat peaches when they are in season." This is excellent advice, though hard to follow for those of you who don't know when peach season is and buy whatever is in the store and have no idea where it came from or when or even what a tree-ripened peach is supposed to taste like.

It was small hardship to give up tomatoes in March, April, May, and June when they really are mush, and high time for me to quit the chorus of Iowa complainers who eat tomatoes in the spring, even though we know better. I already have enough to complain about between Prozac and my hip. Except for pizza and salsa, they were more of a hardship to give up. But I managed.

And that worked too.

But I live in Iowa. And anyone who lives in Iowa can see this next part coming. I knew I couldn't *not* eat tomatoes in summer.

I had to plant tomatoes in my garden, because I live in Iowa. If I didn't plant them in my own garden, church people would stick bags of tomatoes in the back seat of my car if I forgot to lock my car on Sundays. Random strangers might do that on weekdays. So I would eat them in summer. I decided that returning tomatoes to my diet, also eggplant, which I only eat in summer anyway—it's the perfect summer meal along with the tomatoes and sweet corn—would be an experiment to determine if nightshade vegetables did increase my inflammation.

And indeed, they did.

If my pain flared in summer when I was diligent about my stretches and exercise, then maybe it was the tomatoes.

Though it might also be the bed. That's what the lady at the furniture store thinks is wrong with my hip.

Now we have a new bed, and I am going to stop eating tomatoes again, except for when they are in season.

But the pain in my hip has been worse all winter. I usually eat a lot of fiber-rich foods, flaxseed, oatmeal, carrots, broccoli, spinach, some other stuff I don't remember right now, because they are supposed to be anti-inflammatories. But when I had the runs from Prozac, I substituted low-fiber: white bread, white rice, potatoes—all inflammatory. I don't know if that's a proper use for "inflammatory." But it makes me wonder about the relationship between white bread and sugar (also inflammatory) and the level of violence in America. I bet somebody else has already written that book. I know they have used it, sugar that is, as a defense for murder. Remember the "Twinkie defense" in the trial of the guy who assassinated Harvey Milk and Mayor Moscone? Nevertheless, I am pleased with myself for calling Cap'n Crunch "inflammatory."

Except I wish that insight didn't come with so much pain in my hip.

Now my bursitis is back. I have another orthopedic referral, but perhaps you have noticed I am already busy going to doctors and therapists and labs, not to mention Costa Rica, and I haven't had time to make another call. I need a haircut too.

Boy, am I a mess.

And popping ibuprofen like M&M's.

You'd think, if my hip needed heat, that Costa Rica would cure it, like my doctor thought it would cure the runs, and maybe even my depression. Let me pause to give her credit. Costa Rica did cure the runs. Maybe they went away because the Prozac was finally leaving my system. I thought so too. But then they came back for a couple days when I got back to Iowa. Which would support her hypothesis.

Or maybe it's the water, the water in Iowa, that is. You can drink water straight from the tap in Costa Rica. I saw my grandma do it. But not always in Iowa. And you never know in Iowa when it's going to be bad from some hog lot spill or nitrate runoff until you read about it in the paper, which is after you drank the water. I don't get the paper anymore. I buy filtered water instead. So it can't be the water.

Nevertheless, I came home from Costa Rica with a limp. The Voodoo Princess says Costa Rica has "the hardest-ass chairs in the world." The guanacaste is the national tree. It is beautiful, a little like mahogany in color, and durable, and they even make jewelry out of it. But it is hard, hence, "the hardest-ass chairs in the world." The floors also are hard, being mostly tile. If there are wood floors anywhere in Costa Rica, I'm sure they are made of guanacaste, making "hard" and "wood," as in "hardwood floors," a redundancy. By the end of the week, I got shooting pains down my leg as soon as I stepped out of bed.

I don't know how the old people do it. Except none of the Ticos (which is what Costa Ricans call themselves) seem to be old. It turns out appearances are deceiving. Costa Ricans live longer than people in the United States. But they never look old. Most Americans I met in Costa Rica are in their fifties and sixties. I don't think they will live as long as the Ticos, even those who have moved there, because they don't walk. They do not walk. A few take a morning constitutional along the beach. The rest of the day, they drive around in golf carts. The person who sold the golf carts did tell the buyers the carts are not street legal. But I heard the Americans down at the El Bohio puffing indignant because the police confiscated a cart parked in front of the El Bohio and impounded it at the police station across the street where the Americans could see it and drink more beer and get mad all over again. They say the government will have to change the law to make the golf carts street legal, because there are so many of them.

Notice the logic, "There are so many of them." So many illegal golf carts the government will have to make them legal? That's not the way it works in America.

No, "so many of them" must refer to the Americans, not the golf carts. Once you get "so many" Americans in a place, in particular white middle-class Americans who are not used to being the targets of law enforcement, not that anybody besides white middle-class Americans is breaking this particular law, everybody else, even the citizens of the country concerned, will simply have to change to suit the Americans' desires.

You can't escape the Crazy Delusion by sitting on the sofa in your pajamas all day. And you can't escape it by moving to Costa Rica, either.

So I came home from Costa Rica with a limp. How do I answer my coworker's question, "What's wrong with your leg?" Which of these systems would you choose? I choose them all, except maybe the ultrasound machine from the back of the comic book. Each of the others has helped, though none has cured. On the plane ride home, I read an article in the *Wall Street Journal* about an FDA consultation to figure out which of the medications that might be employed to ease the pain in my hip might kill me instead.

Sort of like Prozac.

I wonder how many people on this FDA panel are employed by companies that make these medications? Yes, I will try whatever my doctor prescribes, and will desperately hope it works. But I am getting jaded, have you noticed, about the medical model of poisoning me in the hope of making me well.

I am coming round to the answer my boss gave. It didn't really answer the question. But after all these roundabout ways, it pointed in the direction that I think is the right one: "That's what they used to ask Jacob."

He was talking about the Bible, the book of Genesis: Jacob was returning home to his brother Esau after many years on the lam and was afraid to face him because he had not treated his brother fairly, and Esau had a right to hold a grudge. But he didn't know if Esau still did.

Caroline Myss might weigh in here about being stuck and not being able to move forward. She might tell Jacob to repeat to himself, "I don't need Esau to punish me anymore." But that would enter only partway in, like how the ultrasound never cured the bursitis because it entered only partway in.

Here is what happened next:

> The same night he arose and took his two wives, his two maids, and his eleven children, and crossed the ford of the Jabbok. He took them and sent them across the stream, and likewise everything that he had. And Jacob was left alone; and a man wrestled with him until the breaking of the day. When the man saw that he did not prevail against Jacob, he touched the hollow of his thigh; and Jacob's thigh was put out of joint as he wrestled with him. Then he said, "Let me go, for the day is breaking." But Jacob said, "I will not let you go, unless you bless me." And he said to him, "What is your name?" And he said, "Jacob." Then he said, "Your name shall no more be called Jacob, but Israel [that is, *He who strives with God*], for you have striven with God and with men, and have prevailed." Then Jacob asked him, "Tell me, I pray, your name." But he said, "Why is it that you ask my name?" And there he blessed him. So Jacob called the name of the place Peniel [that is, *The face of God*], saying, "For I have seen God face to face,

and yet my life is preserved." The sun rose upon him as he passed Penuel, limping because of his thigh . . . (Gen. 32:22–31, Revised Standard Version).

For some time now, I have been wrestling with demons. Someday maybe I will write a book about wrestling with angels. Not right now—that subject still scares me. As it should. You really can defeat the demons. But if you can hang onto an angel, in the end you will limp.

Hmm. Maybe Steve, what I call my depression, is an angel. I still wish my hip didn't hurt so much.

A Voice from the Edge

Balancing Act—The Science Chapter

How did I get into this mess, anyway?

Elevated or irritated mood, inflated self-esteem, decreased need for sleep, pressure to keep talking, flight of ideas, distractibility, increase in goal-directed activity, psychomotor agitation, excessive involvement in pleasurable or risky activities—think of these symptoms as a features list, like how a realtor describes a house. They help you decide whether you want to buy, but they are of limited use later when the roof has collapsed.

Why did the roof collapse? The roofer points out there's two feet of snow on it. But there's two feet of snow on the whole neighborhood. And you're the only one being ushered to alternative housing.

It's like this. The original roofer had a bad night, got a little careless in the northeast corner. When the joist got hammered in crooked, it threw off the southeast corner. Things didn't join up. The roofer made adjustments along the line, and the plywood didn't always get centered on the joist. As it turns out, the nails weren't the right size anyway. And they weren't galvanized. Then he ran out of flashing, it was getting late, what harm could that little gap do, the rain comes from the west anyway.

Damn roofer. One issue wouldn't have been a problem. But the more issues there were, the more accommodations had to be made, which created their own anomalies, anomalies not apparent in the half-assed inspection you got before you bought. On the outside, things looked fine.

That's your brain at birth, a little wonky but serviceable. Then, life happened.

Over the years, the roof leaked, not enough to wet the ceiling, which you'd notice, just enough to wet the joists and the ungalvanized nails and start the decay.

You got a little wild there for a while, started throwing rooftop parties, loud music, lots of bass, jumping in unison for some reason you can't remember. Somebody suggested the jumping wasn't good for the roof, but nothing bad ever happened. So it seemed.

However, one day, one week, one damn bitter month, the snow fell. And kept falling. And your roof collapsed. Nobody else's did, but, like I said, you are being escorted to alternative housing.

It's like that.

There is no bipolar bug you could vaccinate against, no poison in the water you could clean up or diet you could adopt, no one gene you could identify in the womb and modify. You might not want to do that anyway. As John McManamy, expert patient and mental health journalist, tells it, the day when lightning struck the log and set it on fire, the Neanderthal who said, "Why don't we drag that thing into this cave and warm up?"— that Neanderthal had bipolar.

You don't want to get rid of this condition. You just want to get a grip.

So, what happened?

In the brain's construction phase, there were some genes that added variety to the plan. One or two would have been fine.

But as the anomalies added up in what would develop into a mind-bogglingly complex network of interacting processes and feedback loops, the potential for breakdown rose.

Next, the brain built pathways between parts and developed those processes and feedback loops. Trying to accommodate its problematic genes, things got wonky.

Throw some environmental factors on top. Your mother's childhood trauma or even her case of the flu while you were riding along in utero counts as an environmental factor. Add a few adverse childhood experiences, maybe somebody who did his/her own jumping on your fragile roof.

Your already wonky brain doesn't have the resilience that other kids' brains have to shake things off. Trace that deficit to genes and environment both. You develop some practices, both neurological and behavioral, to cope. Some of these practices bring short-term benefits but morph into neuroses that will take years of therapy to undo. Others get you into trouble from the get-go. Sleep would soothe the savage beast, but your sleep cycle is one of the wonkier parts of this system, and your impulse control shows it.

So many in the bipolar tribe have what they call comorbid anxiety disorders that anxiety could be considered a key feature of some variants of the condition.[1] The alarm system in your brain may not have a functioning "off" switch. It can dial down within a limited range, but the buzz runs continuously in the background, making you hypersensitive, hyperactive, hyperreactive, which gets you into trouble, creating more trauma, which sets up a cycle that continues to do damage, especially if you start self-medicating to ease the pain.

On the outside, all may be well. In fact, your bursts of activity, properly directed by the appropriate neuroses, may lead to great success, college scholarships, job promotions, friends and influence, lots of parties of which you are the life. Your brain processes information and reaches conclusions with lightning efficiency, and don't ever let your slowpoke psychiatrist forget it. If two feet of snow never falls on your roof, you turn into Christopher Columbus, Teddy Roosevelt, Ted Turner—some astounding if slightly weird overachiever.

However. This is a progressive condition. Each untreated glitch creates another problematic issue, which sets up the next troublesome response, which reinforces a bad pattern, which continues to damage the underlying structure. Until something gives.

Since you can't replace your brain like you can your roof, enter a whole team of doctors, pharmacists, therapists, support groups, websites, and books (see the chapter "Keep Going" in this one) to help you prop it up, develop new habits to reduce the risk of collapse, and house you on those occasions when you need major repairs.

Brain nerds can describe it in one paragraph:[2]

Genes program proteins; proteins make up cells; insert some environmental impact (both internal and external) on how this happens; cells build pathways, which continue to develop; insert some more environmental impact on the direction of development; the brain functions in a particular way, yielding traits that are changeable, or not so much; traits express themselves in behavior; call these behaviors symptoms, if they are the sort that society does not appreciate; insert more environmental impact on the brain's functioning in response to behavior and feedback loops; some behaviors/symptoms are within normal range, and others are diagnosable. Insert the DSM. Or throw it away.

Frederick Goodwin and Kay Jamison wrote *Manic-Depressive Illness*, the bipolar bible, where you can find a more detailed version of this description in head-spinning vocabulary, down to specific locations on DNA strands. They and others who are actually making progress figuring out this disorder say the bottom line has to do with the brain's ability to regulate its responses to a whole range of processes to maintain homeostasis, which is to say, to balance.[3]

That's what went wonky in the developing brain, the capacity to balance.

See, machines are fixed structures. When they work, they do the same thing over and over in a predictable fashion. When they don't work, you fix them. Add some oil, replace a part. Good to go.

Living organisms, on the other hand, continuously grow and respond to changing internal and external environments within a range of measures. Blood pressure, heart and respiration rates, temperature, hormone levels, appetite, energy—that's a short list of measures that rise and fall in response to stimuli, feedback loops, and the time the day.

In a person with bipolar disorder, a whole series of mis-timings and misalignments in our internal and external cycles results in a failure to rebalance.[4] The list includes: *dysregulation* of hormones, neurotransmitters, and immune system; *irregularities* in communication within and between brain cells; and *wonky wiring* among the networks that connect the thinking, feeling, evaluating, and reacting parts of the brain.

Some results are apparent on the surface, affecting mood regulation, cognitive function (attention, working memory, valuing, impulse control), stress response, and circadian (daily) rhythms. Others happen out of sight, including inflammatory activation, cellular and subcellular signaling, energy conversion, metabolism, and brain cell resilience, plasticity, and proliferation.

To make it more interesting, go back to those genes that are implicated, 226 of them and counting. They find new ones all the time. Not all of them are required to get these results. Maybe I have bipolar-related variants in 93; maybe you have variants in 152. We have similar but not identical issues falling under the big bipolar umbrella. Here are some examples of how this plays out for me. You may get a pass on some and have others of your own to add.

Dysregulated neurotransmitters and hormones

Let's start with the most obvious. What goes up must come down. Neurotransmitters are chemicals that carry messages between cells. Dopamine is the up neurotransmitter. Every three years I used to go to the Episcopal Church's national convention, a two-week orgy of committee meetings, Bible studies, worship, parties with buds from seminary, massive legislative sessions, speeches, conflicts, negotiations, and resolutions. Plus a lot of restaurant food. The first meeting would start at 7 a.m., and the last would end around 10 p.m., when I met others to discuss strategy and unwind with a drink. Who needs sleep when it's all so exciting and so *important*?

I was really good at it. My success fed my appetite. I rose to the occasion, in more ways than one. I was bright, charming, energetic, inventive, persuasive, and the life of the party. Hurray for dopamine! Hurray for hypomania! My last convention, a friend who was staying on the same floor of my hotel stopped me at the elevator one morning. She said, "Every time I see you, you're running!"

Then I came home.

That extraordinary amount of dopamine triggered "down-regulation," meaning, enough is enough. So, no more dopamine for me. In its place came two months of depression. After my last convention it was a deep, dark, semipsychotic suicidal depression.

That much, most people know about bipolar.

Dysregulated cortisol makes for less interesting movies but more serious complications healthwise. Cortisol is the get-up-and-go hormone. It gets you out of bed in the morning and manages energy in response to stress.

In a healthy body, cortisol fluctuates throughout the day. Its high morning level gets you out the door on time. An occasional spike when the boss calls you into the office gives you the energy to marshal your resources. By evening, it drops, letting you go to sleep.

If it doesn't drop, if your stress levels are chronic and your cortisol level stays high, you get weight gain, high blood pressure, weak muscles, mood swings, anxiety, fuzzy brain, compromised immune function, poor sleep . . . That pretty much describes my life. How about yours?

In general, healthy means higher in the morning, lower at night. Bipolar means a flattened curve, higher but not quite high enough in the morning, a struggle to get going, and lower but still too high at night, poor sleep followed by a sluggish morning, fuzzy brain causing weak performance at work, raising anxiety level as the day goes on, leading to poor sleep. And repeat.

People with bipolar have a flattened cortisol curve even when not in an episode, not depressed, not manic.[5] This issue could account for much of the lowered life span of those with bipolar. Some of our early death rate comes from increased risk of suicide. But mostly we die from cardiovascular disease and metabolic disorders, often related to this cortisol issue.

Irregularities within and between cells

Here is the cellular piece. There are these little critters inside our cells called mitochondria.[6] They crawled into animal cells at the beginning of animal cells. It is a beautiful relationship, us animals and mitochondria. We provide their nutrients. They in turn run the power plants inside our cells that give us energy to do anything at all, from sparkling at two-week conventions to building new cells inside our brains. The brain uses massive amounts of energy. That's why when mitochondria are in trouble, the brain is too.

My poor pitiful mitochondria weren't up to the task, causing my hippocampus, in charge of memory and mood regulation, to shrink to the size of a pea. At my worst, I lost bills, I lost words, I lost everything my wife said to me on her way out the door in the morning. She took to writing down what I said I would do before she got home, never more than two items. I lost the list.

Wonky wiring among the networks

Meanwhile, tired cells fail to maintain the wiring. One part of the brain really does need to hear from other parts on a regular basis to keep things on an even keel. Like:

My ever-vigilant limbic system told me there was a problem with how my disability benefits were being handled. I brought it to the attention of colleagues who said they would advocate for me. They were friends and exactly the right people for the job. All they needed to do was draw the problem to the attention of the appropriate people, people of goodwill who would surely fix the problem. All I needed to do was wait.

But no. There was a gap between the part of my brain that knew I had done everything I needed to do and the part of my brain that was on full red-alarm alert.[7] No, I didn't need any more documentation. No, I didn't need multiple copies of the documentation. No, I didn't need color-coded sticky notes all over the multiple copies of the several documents. No, I *really* didn't need a map to explain each of the numbered sticky notes. Not one word of this excellent insight from my prefrontal cortex ever crossed my anterior cingulate cortex, in charge of what's a big deal and what isn't, to make its way to my limbic system on red alert to tell it to STAND DOWN.

Finally, my wife took away all the sticky notes, gave me a pill, put me to bed, and worked from home to make sure I stayed there.

By now I was talking about my "Swiss cheese brain." It felt like I had holes in my head. Turns out, I did.

Ventricles

Ventricles are spaces in your brain, like the spaces in your packed suitcase before you press down and squeeze in more stuff. Well, the spaces in your suitcase are filled with air; ventricles are filled with fluid. Everybody has ventricles, the holes where the brain parts (gray matter) and the wires connecting the brain parts (white matter)—aren't.

Dysregulated cortisol burns up brain cells. Oxidative stress on mitochondria means the mitochondria can't power the production of more brain cells. Some of those destroyed-and-not-replaced brain cells are the wiring. The result: bigger holes in my head.

Pay attention, you who think that mania makes you more creative, you who call hypomania an advantage—because who doesn't want to get more work done and be the life of the party? But here's the thing.

The more manic episodes you have, the bigger these holes.[8] Let me repeat that. The more manic episodes you have, the bigger these holes. They've got the pictures, the MRIs to prove it. The bigger the holes, the less you can pack in your suitcase. What you are packing in this suitcase is a functioning brain, which functions less well when there is less of it.

Sheesh! Please don't play around with mania and hypomania. Beyond the mess you get into, it just makes your pitiful brain all the more pitiful.

That was me, 2008–2013, pitiful.

Elevated or irritated mood, inflated self-esteem, decreased need for sleep, pressure to keep talking, flight of ideas, distractibility, increase in goal-directed activity, psychomotor agitation, excessive involvement in pleasurable or risky activities.

That is how the DSM describes mania and hypomania. There are other ways the condition plays out—sleep issues, inflammation, and other cognitive issues that the DSM misses because it is focused on mood and behavior, and our doctors miss because we can still talk a good game—but this gives you an idea. Bipolar disorder has multiple effects throughout a variety of brain systems, both during episodes of depression and mania/hypomania and between episodes. It's not just up and down.

But now you are irritated, because you thought you already knew the answer. It's a chemical imbalance, your friends say, reassuring you it's no big deal, take your meds already. Your brain produces too much or not enough of some mysterious chemical, like how a diabetic pancreas produces not enough insulin. Squirt in some more chemical, good to go.

Nope, not the way it works.

The chemical imbalance theory sets you up, because once you buy the sales pitch and take your pill faithfully every day, you still get sick again. The theory suggests, and everyone who loves you desperately wants it to be true, and really, wouldn't it be nice if it were, that all you have to do is pop your pill, with periodic adjustments when things go bad again.

Wait a minute, did you catch that? If you read the fine print, it says the medication will *reduce* relapse, not eliminate it. Well, there's a bitch, when things go bad again. You, your marriage, your job, your credit rating are at the mercy of this periodic disaster, even if the medication lengthens the gap between disasters. Is it any wonder most people with bipolar have a comorbid anxiety disorder? We live with a piano hanging over our heads, monitoring for the slightest breeze that might mean it's coming down on us.

But that's not the way it works, anyway. It's not that your brain produces too much dopamine, or not enough. It's dysregulation of those chemicals (which sometimes you need more of and sometimes less), pooped cells, and wonky wiring.

Why does it matter how you think of it? Because to fix the problem, or learn to live with it, it helps to understand it.

We can do better when we know what the problem really is. There are tricks to better control the hormones. There are ways to support the cells. There are workarounds to this wiring thing. There are even fixes for the holes. Medication helps, and most people find it essential to keep their life on track. It is one piece of the solution. A big piece, especially on the Bipolar I end of the bipolar spectrum, but only one and not sufficient by itself. I'll get back to the other 499 in the chapter at the end of this book called "Recovery."

OK, grieve. You rolled the genetic dice and came up craps.

But then get over it. Up ahead is Recovery.

You're still in the game.

A Voice from the Edge

Wait, wait! There's More

In April 2013, weeks before the publication of the long-awaited, newly revised DSM-5, Thomas Insel, then director of the National Institute of Mental Health (NIMH) dropped a bomb. In a post written for the NIMH blog, he wrote:

> The strength of each of the editions of DSM has been "reliability"—each edition has ensured that clinicians use the same terms in the same ways. The weakness is its lack of validity. Unlike our definitions of ischemic heart disease, lymphoma, or AIDS, the DSM diagnoses are based on a consensus about clusters of clinical symptoms, not any objective laboratory measure. In the rest of medicine, this would be equivalent to creating diagnostic systems based on the nature of chest pain or the quality of fever . . .
>
> Patients with mental disorders deserve better.[1]

In the post, Insel noted that the increasing genetic and brain-mapping data we have about mental disorders do not match up with the DSM categories. People with different diagnoses have similar genetic markers, and people with the same diagnosis have brains wired differently. The depression junk drawer is not the only example. Some DSM fans conclude that if the data and the diagnoses don't match up, then the objective measures are dead ends, not useful for determining diagnosis and treatment, and irrelevant to the DSM.

Insel's post anticipates the argument:

> Imagine deciding that EKGs were not useful because many patients with chest pain did not have EKG changes. That is what we have been doing for decades when we reject a biomarker because it does not detect a DSM category. We need to begin collecting the genetic, imaging, physiologic, and cognitive data to see how all the data—not just the symptoms—cluster and how these clusters relate to treatment response . . .

Here are examples of what he is talking about, some already known when Insel wrote his post, others being discovered every day:

• Some people with depression do better with antidepressants, some with cognitive behavioral therapy. Generally, which you get depends on how good your insurance is. Your doc would like you to do both to cover your bet and get quicker results, in case the first thing you try doesn't work or makes you crazy. However, one research study, using fMRI, aka functional magnetic resonance imaging (brain scans that reveal when specific parts of the brain are functioning), discovered that the brains of people who do better with medication are wired differently from the brains of those who do better with cognitive therapy.[2] These treatments are not interchangeable. Each works best with a particular wiring.

- fMRIs that record activity in different brain areas at the same time reveal a functional circuit, how the parts work together and which circuits are engaged for a particular task. In one experiment, identifying faces with neutral expressions and faces expressing disgust, people who do not have bipolar engaged the frontal cortex (doing "top-down" processing) while those with bipolar engaged the limbic system ("bottom-up" processing).[3]

- Similar experiments have distinguished between people with bipolar and people with major depression, both while in remission[4] and during a depressive episode.[5]

- Yet another experiment used fMRI and a spatial working memory test to distinguish between people with bipolar and those with ADHD[6], which would be particularly useful when diagnosing children with behavior difficulties whose symptoms make it difficult to distinguish between these two conditions and provide the right treatment in a timely manner.

- Genetic studies reveal that bipolar overlaps more with schizophrenia than with major depression in cortical gene activity.[7] Like the fMRI, genetic testing could steer people away from the wrong med and in the direction of what works for a specific brain dysfunction.

- Even EKGs[8] and blood levels of inflammation[9] have been able to distinguish between people with bipolar and people with major depression. Yes, blood tests.

Some techniques, like genetic testing and brain imaging, have become possible only in recent decades. Some of these biomarkers are relatively new discoveries. They are not "office ready." Don't complain to your doc who isn't using them. Insurance won't pay for them. Complain to your congressperson about NIMH funding.

Insel's point, one of them, is that the new biomarkers don't always match the old DSM categories because *the categories themselves are wrong.*

The DSM puts both major depression and bipolar in the same junk drawer because they share symptoms from the depression menu. But research is demonstrating that the same symptoms do not reflect the same underlying cause. How can we find the underlying cause of a condition that may actually be several different conditions?

It's a chicken and egg issue. We are now developing the possibility of a new classification system that could open up better understandings of mental illnesses and more effective treatments. But we have to use some sort of classification to guide the research. Meanwhile, sick people are sitting in doctors' offices, and doctors are trying to help the best they can with what they've got, which is the DSM's checklists and a handful of pills.

Like Insel says, people with mental illness deserve better. He announced that in the future more NIMH funding will go to projects collecting data to build a new classification of mental disorders.

It's about time.

Which is to say that "Balancing Act" is a good working description of what we know now. At the current rate of funding for brain research, it ought to hold up for at least a decade, maybe two.

But hang in there. More is coming.

Prozac Monologues

Shedding: In which I consider my options

Saturday, February 12, 2005

So. A couple weeks ago, while I was scribbling maniacally during meals, on the plane, at the beginning and end of the day, and all during the middle, Helen was keeping herself busy too. She showed me a list on the plane ride home from Costa Rica. It was a decision tree, laid out like one of those charts you follow, a series of yes or no questions, each answer leading to another question until at the end you find out if you can claim a tax deduction. Or not. In my tax bracket there is little slack in these forms, and the answer is usually "not." I understand in other tax brackets you can get lawyers to find the slack which exists for people who do not earn a living by cleaning houses, or any other way that includes getting up every day and going out the door with a lunchbox.

But Helen's tree was more interesting because the yes or no questions were not about the facts of the matter but rather about what is important. Here is the first question on her decision tree: Could I live outside the country?

Now we are not those people who applied for our passports after the presidential election of 2004. We were already planning to visit Grandma and Mama and the Voodoo Princess and Richie. We even already had the tickets. This is because Helen bought them. She does not put things off, at least not those things that involve searching the Internet to make travel arrangements. This is one of many, many reasons why I have to keep her in my life.

We have often talked about moving to Central America. Helen has lived in Mexico and does mission trips to El Salvador and Honduras. We like the language. We like the people, at least the people who were born there, if not the Americans who came there to smuggle guns in and drugs out. We like the food.

The food is a bigger deal than you might think. When you travel to another country, you might try the local cuisine as part of the travel experience. Actually, the food you eat at the restaurants where tourists feel comfortable drinking the water is not the same as the food your waiter eats at home, even if they have a special section on the menu for *comida típica.* First, you eat a whole lot more of it. Second, you eat more meat. Even if you eat fish, you eat more fish. Nevertheless, if you order the local cuisine, you expand your horizons, which is a good thing.

But when you *live* in another country and shop in the grocery store, that's when the differences really manifest themselves. There are things in the grocery store that you don't know what to do with. And there are things missing from the shelves that you were planning to eat for lunch. It is disorienting to be surrounded by groceries and not know what to eat.

Which is why my mother's meatloaf sells so well. It reminds people who eat it of who they are. The smell of brown gravy and the texture of ground beef on their tongues take them in a time machine back to something called "home" and promise them that if they clean their plate, they can have her chocolate peanut butter cheesecake for dessert. When the smell of cilantro and the sight of butterflies in the grocery aisles tell them they are strangers in a strange land, Meatloaf Monday assures them there are people like them close by, as close as the family table at the Pato Loco.

Now if you have a strong sense of self, you are better able to tolerate being surrounded by people who are not like you. This is one way America is *not* a strong country, and building a wall does not help. It hurts. When you travel, if you spend time with local people, if you learn their ways, eat their food, and especially if you speak their language, you really get to know them and what is important to them; you discover that the people you thought were different from you really are like you after all. And that's good. It expands the space in which you feel at ease, behave well, and generally enjoy life on this wildly diverse and fascinating planet.

But it is still a matter of degree. Even if you become a child of the universe with all its manifold options, it is a conceit to think you didn't bring with you the particular place where you were born. It's not only in the hippocampus; it's all the way into the DNA, and trying to avoid it, for all the posturing, only broadcasts a discomfort you feel inhabiting your own skin. I recommend that you make peace with your skin and what is inside it. Celebrate your own contribution to this wildly diverse and fascinating planet. That is why, if we do move to Costa Rica, you will find us at the Pato Loco, an Italian restaurant, every March 17, eating the *non*-Italian special of the day, corned beef and cabbage, not the pasta dish with the rude name. And after all the paying customers have gone, we will break out the Tullamore Dew, a whiskey distilled down the road from the source of Grandma's DNA, King's County, Ireland.

But you will not find me there on Monday. I know all the expats line up to eat my mother's meatloaf. I ate it most of my childhood, until I learned to make it myself with one ingredient different, and I like mine better. This is called self-differentiation. But much better than any meatloaf at all, I like black beans and rice. So, it would make sense to move to Costa Rica. When we go to the grocery store, we would know what to eat.

Now let's talk about "Shedding." It came from Helen's list, and before that it came from some work I once did on a search committee.

Shedding was a step in a ten-step program. I find it helpful, this process of breaking complex behaviors into manageable steps. The authors of this particular program prefer the word "movement" to the word "step." I think they like movement better than step because they think "step" sounds linear and they prefer to dance. Also, they recognize that to get where you are going, sometimes you have to move backward.

The shortest distance between two points is not necessarily a straight line. Both movement and step could apply to dancing. But step appeals to those who want to march from point A to point B in that straight line. They already know where they are going and how they will get there. You need those people in a group with a task to accomplish, otherwise you never get to point B. Or so it seems. But you also need people who like to dance. Because sometimes everybody agrees to march in a straight line from A to B, but when you get there and turn around, you discover that along the way, a whole lot of people wandered off. Which confuses the people who travel in a straight line because they think their way is easier. It's only easier for them. It's really hard for the people who need to dance. So there you are, or not, if you wandered off along the way.

This process is called "discernment." Some people, the kind who like to dance, eat that word up. But others find it makes their skin crawl. I liked the process but not the word. It made my skin crawl. This was before I ever took Prozac; it wasn't a side effect from going off it. If it makes your skin crawl, or if you don't know what the heck I am talking about, here is a definition for both the dancing and the marching people. Discernment means figuring out, when you do it with your gut as well as your head. With your heart, as well, as long as you also use your head. Discernment is figuring out, using all your systems. When you do it in a group, you bump up against all the different ways people dance or march to get somewhere. To do it well in a group, then your need to get everybody else to move the way you move is one of the things you need to shed. In my experience, the people who like to dance have just as hard a time shedding this need as the people who like to march.

The shedding step was a question each person on the search committee answered, "What do I need to give up to seek just one thing, what God yearns for in this decision?"

Well, clearly, to put the question in these words presumes the one thing you want is God's will. I won't presume that for you, or even claim that our decision-making about Costa Rica has been framed in that way.

Helen didn't like the shedding step in the search committee. She was afraid I would shed something important to her. She was going to be affected by the decision, but she wouldn't get a say about it because she wasn't on the committee. But she likes the word now, because she reframed the question. Her way of framing it might help you, when you are making a major decision, like about moving to Costa Rica, even if you don't bring the God thing into it.

She asked, "What can I *not* shed?" Put another way, "What do I need to *keep*, and if I had to give it up in order to move to Costa Rica, then I won't move to Costa Rica?"

Can you see how that might be a useful question when you have a decision to make? Take out the words "move to Costa Rica" and fill in your own decision, like "take this new job" or "get a dog," things like that, which inevitably lead to changes in all the rest of your life, whether you are paying attention to that reality when you make the decision or you ignore it until later when it bites you in the butt.

She showed me her list of what she would *not* give up, or shed, to move to Costa Rica. There were four items. And I was the first one.

Now given what a mess I have been lately, and how many dishes she has washed, which is not her favorite chore and I used to do it, plus putting away the laundry which is not my favorite so she did that already, and how much time I spent by myself scribbling on a yellow notepad while we were on vacation in Costa Rica and even the seven and a half hours on the plane *each way* when she didn't have anywhere else to go or anyone else to talk to, this was most gratifying.

After me came Mazie the Wonder Dog, the blue bowl, and our new bed. OK, it's not that there is a deep emotional attachment to this piece of furniture. But we put down major bucks on the thing before we left for Costa Rica and it wasn't delivered until last week after we got back. Helen wasn't prepared to let go of it until she got to sleep on it. There *is* a deep emotional attachment to the blue bowl. But I came first, and then Mazie.

I thought it was a most excellent list, and an indicator that we might be able to pull this move off.

Helen's list got me to think about my own list. I didn't try to answer the shedding question because I don't trust my brain right now. But I broke it down for myself:

Could I shed my bird feeder?

Could I shed sweet corn?

Could I shed fireflies?

When I shared my list with friends at dinner, they jumped all over the bird thing. There are 868 species of birds in Costa Rica. They thought surely, I would find new birds, even if they didn't need me to feed them. Well, there are hundreds of dogs in

Playas del Coco. Nevertheless, we couldn't move to Costa Rica if it meant giving up Mazie the Wonder Dog. I mean, this is a dog who waits for us to say grace before she eats.

None of the birds in Costa Rica will ever wait for me to say grace and pour a cup of birdseed into a feeder every morning, the blend with extra sunflower seeds because our cardinals like it. Not "our cardinals" in the possessive sense. We don't own these cardinals. More like in the sense of our cousins or our neighbors. Mama Cardinal, Daddy Cardinal, and Old Cardinal. Francis of Assisi would say, Sister Cardinal, Brother Cardinal. Plus, a number of finches and sparrows, and the condominium where they all live in the arbor vitae at the end of the deck. I don't know if we will ever have "our" kiskadees, with a connection that crosses the boundary of species. A few other boundaries, too, now that I mention it, genus, family, order. We do share class and kingdom. I might not be quite as attached if we didn't, because I am not Francis. Sister Stinging Ant? I'm not there, yet.

We never got to sweet corn at the dinner table when my friends objected to my attachment to my bird feeder. So, I will continue the discussion with you. If you live in Iowa, you already understand that in Iowa, sweet corn is a sacrament.

I loved corn on the cob when I was a little girl growing up in Colorado. But it may as well have been canned. It's a different vegetable outside of Iowa. It's one of those "enhancing the quality of your life" issues I was talking about earlier. Remember—only eat peaches in season? But it's not just the season. It's the geography. Because the timing of sweet corn is exceedingly short.

Here is how you prepare Iowa sweet corn as a sacrament:

1. Come to Iowa in late July, to a house with a patch of sweet corn in the backyard.
2. Prepare everything else for dinner and have it waiting on the table.

3. Put a big pot of water on to boil.

4. Once the water is boiling AND NOT BEFORE, go out to the backyard and pick the corn.

5. Shuck the corn on the way back into the house, dropping the husks and silks on the grass as you go. If you are cooking for a crowd, each person should shuck his/her own ear. It's too hard to shuck while carrying more than three ears, one in your hands and one tucked into each armpit. And once you have shucked one of the three ears, you really don't want to put it back into your armpit so you can shuck the next ear anyway. Not in Iowa in July. No, it really is best for each person to shuck his/her own ear.

6. Put the corn in the boiling water.

Now the great debate begins, and I won't express a dogmatic opinion on the subject. Which indicates I grew up in Colorado, not Iowa, or else I *would* be dogmatic on this point. People native to Iowa have firm opinions on the question, How long? I used to boil my sweet corn for two minutes. Now I do it for ten. I can't remember why. At the risk of incurring the wrath of Iowa, I will say, do what you like.

Some people add salt to the water. Some people add sugar. Others positively disapprove of the sugar and insist it is clinging to old, outdated ways because sweet corn has been bred lately to be even sweeter than it used to be. I do have an opinion about that one. Save the sugar for field corn. Or for the stuff you had to buy at the grocery store, because the raccoons took your entire crop this year, and the truck on the corner parking lot ran out early today.

Butter, salt, pepper, chili powder—these are all matters of personal taste. Even in Iowa we allow this sort of variation and enjoy discussing the options. I eat mine naked as the day it was born. Please do not use margarine. As Paul Prudhomme taught my mother to say when she was in his cooking school, I will not meet my Maker with margarine on my breath. It would be a shame for you to choke on the sweet corn and suddenly find yourself in front of the Judge of the quick and the dead, dead in this case, with clear evidence on your breath that you have not properly honored God's good creation because you put margarine on sweet corn.

Sweet corn made its way into national news during the last presidential election. Because Iowa was a contested state, the president came to Iowa and took a bite out of an ear that wasn't cooked at all. If the incident raised a question in your mind, let me assure you. Sweet corn is good even raw. I break the ears in half so I can use a smaller pot and nibble a few kernels before dropping them into the water. But this is Iowa, not Texas. We tolerate somebody who bites into sweet corn raw. Many of us even voted for somebody who did that. But we don't think it's a sign of manliness. More like poor impulse control. In Iowa, poor impulse control is not the same as manliness, though it seems to be in Texas.

Sweet corn has become part of who I am inside my skin. Corn is sacred in the southwestern part of the United States. But it's a different kind of corn. Same genus, different species. I don't know if it's sacred in Costa Rica. Sugarcane seemed to be the big deal when we were there. They were burning fields in preparation for harvest. Before sugarcane, cattle were the big deal. I don't know if cattle were sacred. Cowboys are important, and it's not only for the tourists. Having lived both in Colorado and in Iowa, I know that cattle and sweet corn are *vastly* different cultures. Those two cultures even fought a war, the Range War in the late nineteenth century. We're still not quite over it.

Iowa means "beautiful land," and I am connected to that land, like I am connected to our cardinals. So it's something to think about.

Then there are the fireflies. I once turned down a job that would have been a promotion and much bigger salary, plus health insurance, which I didn't have at the time, because I couldn't let go of the fireflies. The job was in New Jersey. Which did have something to do with it. Sorry, New Jersey. The person who offered me the job said they have fireflies in New Jersey. I know New Jersey is the Garden State, and there are farms. I believed him that there are fireflies. I sort of believed him. I would have to see for myself, before I took a job in New Jersey.

But I couldn't believe there are fireflies in Newark, which is where the job was. And I couldn't bring myself to work in Newark but live in the suburbs, any more than I could move to Costa Rica but live in the compound where all the people drive their golf carts. I just think you might as well stay home. And eat canned corn.

Here's the thing about things. If you can't let go of them, then you don't own them. They own you. It seems to me that birds and sweet corn and fireflies are too lovely and too good to deserve my turning them into chains. But they are a part of who I am, and they do feed my soul. I have to figure out whether they can feed my soul from a distance, whether the place inside my skin and the place my skin is in have to be the same place, or if they can be different.

But there was a little girl born in Drumright, Oklahoma, in 1911, and today she sits in her wheelchair at the family table in Playas del Coco, Costa Rica. She has shed many things in her lifetime, some quite precious to her, to bring her to that beautiful place. And I am her beloved grandchild. If her freedom of spirit is in my own DNA, then maybe I can shed a few things too.

Prozac Monologues

Pura Vida: In which I choose life

Tuesday, February 15, 2005

My therapist tells me I need to finish my writing because the depression is fueling the writing, and I won't let go of it until I finish. Or something like that. She was taking the notes, not me.

I've seen her a couple of times now since I got back to Iowa. I watch her as carefully as she watches me. She's a cheerful person. She greets me with a smile in the waiting room and asks, "How are you?" When I hesitate, she answers for me, "We'll find out, won't we," then laughs at her own joke, invites me into her office, sits in her rocking chair, picks up her notebook and pen, and looks up at me with attention. She seems to hear what I say better than I do. Words come out of my mouth, and she pays more attention to them than I do. I can enjoy her cheerfulness and not feel misunderstood, not like "If she really understood me, she would be depressed too." She doesn't smile at my bizarre thoughts, which helps me feel understood, even though I smile when I tell them. I think they are funny. Sometimes. I am tired of having them. At least sometimes.

I wonder how this therapy thing will go. I have resisted it for so long, ever since my last therapist's notes were subpoenaed for the custody hearing. The notes were never used, but still.

I told her people say her middle name is "Not-For-Wimps." She nodded. Evidently, she already knew. Maybe she gave herself the name. She said, "That's only for those who don't try. The other day somebody came in whining because he got fired for coming to work drunk. I said, 'What did you expect?'"

Jacob got a taste of Not-For-Wimps a few years ago when we were seeing her for family therapy. He was feeling teenaged put upon. So he said the kind of self-delusional self-defense thing one says when feeling put upon. Not-For-Wimps responded, "Everybody who does not believe a single word Jacob just said, raise your hand." And three hands, Helen's, mine, and Not-For-Wimps's, shot into the air.

For now, my therapist smiles when she greets me, but not when I talk about my plan. I like these things about her, even though I did not like it when the drive-by doctor did not smile when I joked about my plan. I think that means I am moving to a new place. Caroline Myss, whose book said I can heal myself, would expect my hip to stop hurting soon. Though I don't expect my depression to yield to an affirmation.

When I have sat in the other chair, on the other side of the helper/helped relationship, it didn't depress me to listen to somebody else's pain. It made me feel honored, enormously honored. People's stories are sacred, when they really tell them, instead of telling you what they think you want to hear.

It's hard to believe in the sacredness of your story when you don't like your story and when it's about pain. But if it is the truth, it comes from God, even if it is about pain.

Costa Rica has its own take on this issue, *pura vida*.

Everywhere we went, we saw the phrase *pura vida*. It seems

to be the country's motto, in newspapers and travel brochures, on T-shirts and ball caps. It's an interesting way for a country to present itself to visitors. Compare it to "God Bless America." People say *pura vida* to each other when they mean they are happy to do the favor you asked, that they share your gladness for your good news, that some minor inconvenience is really part of the joy of living, or even a major inconvenience, that they live in Costa Rica. Isn't it an incredible sunset, meal, or mud puddle. *Pura vida.*

Helen is the fluent Spanish speaker. I am still at the stage of starting conversations I cannot finish. She explained *pura vida* to me. She said at first she thought *vida pura* would be better grammar. In Spanish the noun (*vida* means life) comes first, then the adjective (*pura* means pure). Then she realized if they said *vida pura*, it would mean "a pure life." But the other way, *pura vida* means simply "pure life," or "life to the full, life in its abundance." They are not the same. Do you get it? When you speak another language, you have to use the thought patterns of that language. And *pura vida* is the way people in Costa Rica think.

Consider what the words mean in their absence. What if you didn't have *vida pura*—a pure life? Then you would have a life that is not pure, a life that doesn't measure up in the purity department. And there you go, trying to figure out which part of life is pure and which part is not. *Vida pura*, a pure life, hooks you into a certain habit of thought, the habit of thinking about which things ought to be and which things ought not to be.

But if you don't have *pura vida*—pure life—then what you do have is a life diminished by concerns that draw you *from* life, like thinking about which things ought not to be. *Pura vida* invites you to embrace the fullness that is right in front of you. And that habit of thought is about what is, simply is.

To be or not to be—that was how Hamlet put the suicide question. I don't remember if he had a plan. But it seems to me he spent a lot of time "not being," even before he got himself killed. He didn't exactly embrace life, which made it hard for him to get over his depression.

Does it disturb you to know that I am a priest? So many people jump to conclusions when they get that information. Do you wonder whether I *should* be a priest, on account of whether you think my life is pure? Or not? Whether a priest should have these bizarre thoughts of mine? Or not? Whether a priest should acknowledge them out loud? Or not?

If it helps, I will say yes, I do believe some things are sinful, and I try not to do them. But that is not what my story is about, and I won't waste any more thought on that issue. The track I am on is *pura vida*.

Along with Moses, I choose life.

All of it, the life that was created and is cherished by the One whose name is I AM WHO I AM. "Thus you shall say to the Israelites, 'I AM has sent me to you'" (Exod. 3:14, New Revised Standard Version).

I am too. This whole story is. It just is. And life will win, even if all that energy I had in Costa Rica has run down and I am tired now.

My mother gets a kick out of having a priest in the family. When I was pregnant with Jacob, she got to tell her friends, "My daughter, the Father, is going to be a mother." Oh well. I am learning to embrace my own obnoxious mother side. I can embrace hers too. She is Catholic. I don't think she really believes that having a child who is a priest will earn her any brownie points on the way to heaven, on account of she gave one of hers back to God. Maybe she does. But I am an Episcopal priest. There isn't the celibacy thing to rack up the major points. Nevertheless, a priest in the family comes in handy for the miscellaneous ritual. So she invited me to Costa Rica to bless the bar.

We blessed the bar right before its grand opening. I called

it a bar mitzvah, which confused the people who knew anything about Judaism. This is what the dictionary says: "mitzvah (a) a Biblical or rabbinic commandment; (b) an act of charity performed in the interests of the Jewish religion or law, or of any individual." And a *bar* mitzvah is when a Jewish boy becomes a man by taking upon himself the responsibility of the Law.

So "mitzvah" doesn't exactly mean "blessing." I was being poetic. That said, Moses was clear that the commandments were a blessing, and all the Wisdom literature agrees, and so do the rabbis. And among the commandments, "Choose life" is surely one that blesses.

Maybe you know the Big Ten, the ones that get carved on rocks and put in front of courthouses to remind us all that without the divine revelation of the Old and New Testaments, we would be a bunch of savages with no law and America would cease to be a great nation, even though there were lots of laws and lots of cultures that carved their laws into rocks long before Moses ever got around to the Big Ten. I will believe the people who put the Ten Commandments up in public places are serious about them when they put the last one, *Thou shalt not covet thy neighbor's goods*, on placards and picket the shopping malls. In other words, when they really address the Crazy Delusion instead of using their righteousness to distract us from it.

There are 613 commandments in the Torah. Jesus said two of them summed up the rest. The first comes from Deuteronomy, "Hear, O Israel, the LORD is our God, the LORD alone. You shall love the LORD your God with all your heart, and with all your soul, and with all your might" (Deut. 6:4–5, NRSV). The second comes from Leviticus, "You shall love your neighbor as yourself" (Lev. 19:18, NRSV). Moses got them down to one. It's not counted as one of the 613. But it's the last thing he said about the subject, and it summed up everything that went before, Deuteronomy 30:19, "Choose life." In Hasidism, the Eastern European branch of Judaism that keeps the Law the strictest and dances the wildest, if there is ever any competing claim in any particular situation, *Choose life* is the commandment that trumps any of the 613. Surely it must be the greatest blessing.

Choose life is a mitzvah in the first sense, a Biblical or rabbinic commandment. Helping somebody who is depressed to choose life is a mitzvah in the second sense, "an act of charity performed in the interests of the Jewish religion or law, or of any individual." And both are a blessing. That is why I called my bar blessing a bar mitzvah. I think the rabbis would like my reasoning. Some of them would. At least they would be amused.

Here is what happened at our bar mitzvah, January 26, 2005:

The Voodoo Princess and Richie, Mama, three guests at the hotel, and Helen and I stood at the bar. Grandma, as always, was seated. It's a small bar, room for half a dozen to lean against it, eight if they are really friendly. It is made of white tile, lovely really, and exactly high enough for the Voodoo Princess to lean against it on her elbow. That's how they determined the height when they built it, so she could lean against it on her elbow. Sort of like using Pharaoh's foot to decide how long a foot was.

My mother read the Scripture passage. It was the passage we picked for my stepfather's funeral, and she wants it at her funeral too. "On this mountain the LORD of hosts will make for all peoples a feast of fat things, a feast of wine on the lees, of fat things full of marrow, of wine on the lees well refined" (Is. 25:6, RSV).

Can you see how it would be my mother's favorite, since she thinks butter is a sacrament and margarine is a sin? Isaiah was a prophet who had visions of heaven. You'd expect him to know, and my mother is counting on it. There will be butter in heaven.

This was (approximately) my sermon:

"I couldn't find a liturgy for a bar blessing in my reference books. But a trained liturgist knows the principles. An object is blessed and is a blessing, or is cursed and is a curse by the use to which it is put. That is readily apparent when we are talking about a bar. If a bar is used to celebrate life, then it is blessed and it is a blessing. If it is used to hide from life, then it is cursed and it is a curse.

"I found a cross that conveys this concept. Jesus is alive on this cross, his hands stretching to reach into the night on the left and the day on the right, the background filled with the sun, the moon, the stars, birds, fruits, flowers. See the bats perched on his left arm? Did you know there are 108 different species of bats in Costa Rica?

"At first, I thought it was the Christ of the Fourth Day of Creation, sun, moon, and stars. But then I realized, it's the Christ of *Pura Vida*, pure life. God reaches into all of it, the darkness as well as the light.

"May this bar not be used to hide from the darkness, because that would be hiding from the part of life that is dark. And you would miss the part of God's embrace that reaches to you only in the darkness. May this bar celebrate all of life."

Then my acolyte—that's "bartender" in the language of Episcopalians—popped the cork on the champagne bottle and poured nine paper cups of champagne, even one for Grandma. Yes, Grandma took the Pledge in Oklahoma as a little girl, but it seems to be wearing out. Isaiah promised there will be wine in heaven. And she's getting ready. We spilled a bit of the champagne on the bar, and everybody rubbed it in as well as you can rub champagne into tile. Then we lifted our glasses and toasted, *Pura vida!*

That's how to bless a bar. If you are a priest and the occasion arises, now you have a liturgy.

Christ of *Pura Vida* now hangs at the bar. If you go to the Pato Loco, you can look up at him and contemplate the bats resting on his arm as you sip your Imperial and chat with the Voodoo Princess.

One of the guests said she was moved by what I said about the embrace of God in the dark, and she gave me her copy of

St. John of the Cross's *Dark Night of the Soul*. Thomas Moore wrote a book about depression that he called *Dark Nights of the Soul*. Sometimes people talk about their own dark night like it's their midlife crisis or a sleepless night from a bad conscience. But St. John of the Cross lived a long time ago, before midlife crises and self-help books. I have heard of his book. I thanked this lady for it, but I don't think I will read it right away. It is a book for the stout of heart, and I don't know if I am up to it.

Spirituality is like cooking. Some people like to read recipes. Some people like to eat. I always wonder, when people want to talk with me about spirituality, which of these they are.

When it comes to cooking, I like to do both, read and eat. But I prefer to eat. When it comes to spirituality, I would rather read a murder mystery. Maybe *Dark Night of the Soul* will illumine my darkness. But not today. Today my plate is full.

So now it is time to take my new medications, talk to my therapist, walk Mazie the Wonder Dog, time to love, to learn, to touch, to live. I feel sadder than when I was in Costa Rica. But then I felt crazier. I prefer where I am now. It was a roundabout way, this whole trip. There may be a few more twists in the road ahead. But I know I am starting to move in the right direction. Don't feel sad for me.

Even if you feel sad for yourself right now, even if you can't believe a word I am saying, I will say it anyhow.

You are not alone. Even in the darkness, you are not alone. Choose life.

A Voice from the Edge

Recovery

Sure, and wouldn't that have been an excellent place to end, *Choose life*?

Everybody loved the ending of my last monologue. It made my therapist smile. Over the next few years I worked hard to make my therapist smile. It's not a good thing to do, by the way, try to make your therapist smile. That's why the doc refused to smile when I said I didn't "plan to use my plan." The effort wastes the session. You're supposed to spend the time saying what you can't say anywhere else. But everywhere else, people love it when you say things to make them smile. They want you to get better, and rare is the person who can resist reinforcing any behavior on your part that deceives them into thinking you are.

I wasn't getting better. I was sliding in and out of mixed episodes, mild psychosis, and not-so-mild suicidality as I kept trying yet another antidepressant.

Yada, yada, yada. Six antidepressants, three sledgehammer sleep aids (utterly useless), a fistful of augmentation strategies, and one benzo later, I began to believe the results of the MDQ and finally told my third psychiatrist.

I had been off the medication ranch for over a year after I quit The Feedbag. But in 2008 when I was going under again, Helen appealed to a colleague in the psychiatry department where she worked. He appealed to another colleague who was not taking new patients. But she took me. I call her The Winner.

Finally, a psychiatrist who respected me, who knew I had a brain, had done my research, and could speak her language. We had real conversations about her recommendations. Now initially she made the same call as the others, major depression, and we started by repeating an antidepressant that had the virtue of never having taken me to the edge. It hadn't worked the last time I took it. But it was a generic, and The Feedbag didn't give it much of a chance before switching me to a pricier alternative. After a genuine trial this time, we decided the generic really didn't work after all, which is when I mentioned the MDQ and raised the possibility that the diagnosis was wrong. We could be looking at Bipolar II.

The Winner was dubious—I never exhibited "up" in her office—until Helen came to an appointment with me and told her about how I wrote a book in a week while on vacation in Costa Rica. Hypomania for more than four days ticked the last box.

Funny thing, I knew in my head that my manic writing was a symptom of bipolar, in fact, the very symptom we were explaining to The Winner at the appointment. Nevertheless, that day and whenever Helen describes how startled she was, and scared, to be sitting next to this driven stranger I had suddenly become, lost in my yellow legal pad, oblivious to her efforts to gain my attention, I still believe Helen was making an awfully big deal out of it.

That's when I got a new diagnosis, Bipolar NOS (Not Otherwise Specified). NOS is now called "Unspecified" in the DSM-5. Whatever. The code hedges the bet and seems to be the diagnosis preferred by psychiatrists who recognize the spectrum, that bipolar doesn't divide into distinct categories but rather manifests across a range of symptoms somewhere between the clear-cut symptom silos of Bipolar I and major depressive disorder. That's not exactly what the DSM-5 intends by "Unspecified," but it is a way of letting the psychiatrist explore not *Do you have bipolar?* but rather *How* much *bipolar do you have?* Now, with some kind of bipolar diagnosis, we had new, less dangerous strategies to pursue.

Meanwhile, I had started a blog, *Prozac Monologues: Reflections and Research on the Mind, the Brain, Mental Illness, and Society.*

The blog helped.

It focused my own research into the burning question, *What the hell happened to my brain?*

It provided cognitive rehabilitation, as my drug-addled and cognitively damaged brain struggled to put words together for a few paragraphs each week.

It introduced me to other bloggers, other people with mental illness, and even an occasional doctor who made comments.

It kept me from feeling invisible once I was on disability and wasn't going to two-week conventions or much of anywhere else anymore.

It restored my sense of worth, which had been battered by going on disability.

It was fun. It had been a long time since I had any fun.

Through my blog, I found John McManamy's blog, *Knowledge Is Necessity*. And through John, I found the research of Sarah Russell at the University of Melbourne, Australia. Russell interviewed one hundred patients with bipolar who had stayed symptom-free and behaving normally for two years, or at least had a sense of control over their illness. They ranged from eighteen to eighty-three years old. Seventy-six percent were in paid employment. Thirty-eight percent were raising children.

She asked, "What do you do to stay well?" A Canadian study later replicated her findings. Both found the same strategies:

- Lifestyle
- Education and self-awareness
- Support
- Medication

In that order.

Now, understand me. This list is not how you get out of your alternative housing after the roof falls in. It is how people who are stable stay stable, more or less. It is how I stay stable, more or less. Catch the recovery train, do your best to stay on it. When you fall off, do what you need to do to get back on it, and do your best again to stay on it. The more you do it, the easier it gets, even if it never actually gets easy. This is Recovery. And this is the rest of my life.

Lifestyle

Sleep, diet, exercise, stress management, including meditation and reflection—these are the foundations for recovery.

And the greatest of these is sleep.

My inner clock is wonky. Maybe yours is too. All those different hormones that tell us when it is time to be awake, sleepy, hungry, energized, anxious, calm, warm, and cool operate in relation to each other like gears of a clock. When the clock gets bumped, daylight savings time, a late-night party, a change in work schedule, the brain readjusts. But not the bipolar brain. The bipolar brain pops a gear.

Ellen Frank invented Interpersonal Social Rhythms Therapy (IPSRT) to put the clock in a shock-absorbing case. There are a number of events that set and reset the clock throughout the day. The basic idea of IPSRT is this: make sure these events happen at the same time every day. Frank first identified seventeen daily events to track on a big chart. Then she got real. Can you track seventeen points in your schedule on a daily basis? If so, you may have a mental illness, but it's not bipolar! It turns out five of the seventeen give the most bang for your buck anyway: out of bed, first contact with another person, start work/school/family care, dinner, back to bed.

When I started this, I was in tears from the effort to track even two, when I got in and out of bed. But those two set up the others, so there you go. Make your own chart. Track those two times. Add another, first contact with another person, if you can manage it. Track your moods. After a month, look for a correlation between the regularity of your schedule and the regularity of your moods.

That is the social rhythms part. The interpersonal part is plain old therapy addressing whatever issues prevent you from protecting your clock. Does a fight with your spouse keep you twirling at night so you oversleep the next morning? Learn better skills to resolve your differences. Does your lack of education keep you stuck in shift work and a constantly changing schedule? Address the lack of confidence that derailed your schooling and get back at it. Has your disability taken away your go-to-work-time prompt? Explore your interests and motivation and find something else to do at a set time.

Like that.

Bottom line: sleep is your friend. It is the reset button on your brain. Seriously, sleep is when your brain takes out the neurological trash. All those articles about how to get a good night's sleep, read them. Do what they say.

Here is my sleep hygiene: I eat my big meal at lunch, and a light meal for supper; I don't drink coffee after 2 p.m.; I turn off work, Facebook, and email at 5 p.m.; I limit alcohol, and none after 7 p.m.; I wear amber glasses after 8 p.m. to filter out the blue light that tells the pineal gland to wake up, and a mask in bed to block out the smoke alarm light and, God help us, the full moon; I keep the bedroom cool; I try to remember the mind tricks my therapist teaches me to shut down the late-night mental motor vehicle spinning its wheels in mud. I turn down a lot of dinner parties that would overstimulate me at night. Not perfectly, especially the mind tricks part, I suck at mind tricks, but that's my program.

If I get off track and don't get enough sleep for three nights in a row, I take a rescue med, something taken occasionally as needed. Three sleepless nights send me into an anxious depression, which then sets its own rhythm. Then I get angry, hopeless, have a double martini, wine with dinner, a chocolate dessert . . . *To hell with these restrictions.* Things go downhill from there. *To hell with therapy, it's not working anyway, my therapist is plotting to put me in the hospital, is this the rest of my life, haven't I lived long enough already . . .*

I try to reset my clock before it comes to that.

The rest of this lifestyle stuff, diet, exercise, stress management, including meditation and reflection—you know what to do. Just do it!

OK, in the throes of an episode, this stuff is impossible. Taking a shower is impossible. I know. I'm not here to beat you up for what you can't do.

Use your remissions. When you are able, pick one self-care strategy. Just one. Baby steps. Babies fall down a lot when they are learning to walk, and you will too. But each step makes the next one more possible.

For example—sugar. I learned to eat right thirteen years ago, and do a pretty good job, lots of fruit and veggies, whole grains, fish, beans, unprocessed and organic as much as possible. Healthy food makes for happy mitochondria makes for healthy brain.

Sugar is not a major food group for me, a piece of See's after lunch, a package of Peeps at Easter, just one, a shared dessert when I go out.

Sugar—it's poison, I know. It screws up the GABA/glutamate balance.[1] Those are the stop and go hormones in your brain.[2] When I combine sugar with coffee and red wine, I can feel the glutamate hormones flooding my body. Go, go, go

. . . no particular destination, mostly it's my cells banging their heads against the wall. Thirteen years I have been eating right. Over thirteen years, I have adopted almost every single bipolar self-care strategy out there except journaling (long story), eliminating alcohol altogether, and no sugar.

Then last year my energy level plummeted after a different long illness and hasn't fully returned. Nevertheless, I still want to walk the Camino someday—five hundred miles across northern Spain to Santiago de Compostela. I need my energy back. Now I had two reasons to give up sugar. The time had come for my first Peep-less Easter.

On top of everything else this condition has taken from me, now no Peeps for Easter? Damn, I hate bipolar.

One step at a time. If it takes you ten years before you get outside the house to take a walk, well, after thirteen years I am almost but not quite clean of sugar.

The lifestyle issues are the hardest, the absolute hardest. We're talking lifelong behaviors. That in itself is hard, especially when none of these is the magic bullet. But each one helps. One helps 10 percent, another 30 percent, another 3 percent. They add up, even the 3 percent behavior, and as they do, your stability increases. As your stability increases, it is easier to tackle other behaviors.

The real bitch is, nobody else around you has to change, and many are actively subverting your efforts. OK, sure, half the people around you need to eat better. But if they don't, they aren't hauled off to alternative housing. So, when they put cake in front of you, tell *them* to eat it. You eat a handful of nuts or a couple dates instead. Fight for yourself, your health, your life.

One more lifestyle item that offers big bang for your buck—controlled breathing. It's the best anti-anxiety drug out there, it's free, immediately available, and has no side effects. A slow intake on a count of five, all the way to your belly, hold for a count of three, a slow release for seven. And repeat.

Advanced breathing adds mindfulness. Get quiet. Breathe. Pay attention to your breath. When something distracts you, note it and refocus on your breath. When your mind wanders—it will wander, of course it will wander—note it, refocus on your breath. Over and over. Don't worry about how often your mind wanders. This is a meditation *practice*. Every time you refocus, you are doing another rep. The more reps, the stronger your brain gets.

Do this on a semiregular basis. The meditators out there will tell you every day, same time of day, some ridiculous amount of time. Sure. I do it once in a while for a few minutes. I consider three minutes before I give up a victory. My brain is unruly. I know the breath meditation would tame my unruly brain. But part of my self-care is to reject perfectionism. That's my story and I'm sticking to it.

The lifestyle changes are your best strategies for regulating those dysregulated hormones, cortisol, GABA, and glutamate, and for keeping your mitochondria happy, strengthening cells. I spent more time on lifestyle here than I will on the other strategies because, repeat after me: lifestyle is the foundation to recovery . . . and the greatest of these is sleep.

Education and Self-Awareness

The more you know about your wonky brain, the better equipped you are to deal with it.

What I knew about medication protected me from The Feedbag. I knew not to start an addictive antidepressant right before I left for a five-week stay in Costa Rica back in 2006, in case it was a mistake and I would need her help to taper off it, which it was, and I did, five weeks later after I got back. I wish I had known she should have been monitoring my liver status, because she didn't, and that caused problems my fabulous family practitioner caught, but not until months later. I was still learning.

When I learned what the bipolar experts say about antidepressants, I realized why I had to fully disclose to The Winner, so she could prescribe the right medications, not the wrong ones.

When I learned all the nonmedication tricks, I had a foundation to keep me going when the medication tricks didn't.

When I could ask informed questions, The Winner and I could explore alternatives together, which improved the quality of my care. In the middle of our discussion about something she was recommending, she once told her resident, who was observing the appointment, "This is not a good example of how you discuss medication with a typical patient." We were using technical words. We were referring to research. You don't have to be a typical patient either. You can bring real information to the table.

Oh, and one of the coolest benefits of education happens inside your brain where you can't even see. Learning stimulates BDNF, brain-derived neurotrophic factor.[3] This little gem of a protein stimulates the brain to create more brain cells. It patches those holes in my head! It works especially well in partnership with the healthy mitochondria I now have because I eat oatmeal sweetened by raisins instead of Cap'n Crunch for breakfast.

Then there is the self-awareness piece. Russell found that people who do well are microscopically attuned to triggers and early shifts in mood or energy. Way before their doctors ever notice, they take action themselves. For me that means knowing when I can go to the party or take on another responsibility, and when I need to dial it back; when controlled breathing and a brisk walk are adequate to control my anxiety, and when I need a rescue med; when my three little ounces of wine with dinner are fine, and when a creeping depression suggests I abstain for a while.

The other piece is educating others. *Isn't everybody a little bit bipolar? Oh, come on, what would* [fill in the blank] *hurt this once? Are you sure you still need medication?* We could come up with a long list of ignorant things that ignorant people tell us, couldn't we.

Most of these people genuinely care about us and want to help. Most of them. When we are educated about our condition, we can give them information that could make their help more helpful. And we can recognize and reject the nonsense.

Support

In 1984, Jacob's father and I were touring Midwest zoos, the last big vacation we'd take before having to haul along all the baby paraphernalia. In the St. Louis Zoo, we came across a pen demonstrating an experimental procedure to save an endangered species of zebra. Using in vitro fertilization, the vets implanted zebra embryos in horses, who carried the baby zebras to term. Which meant a zebra could produce more eggs and more than one baby in a year, while not enduring the risk of labor.

There was a newborn, in all its striped glory, leaning against mama palomino's haunch, while its gaze was fixed on the next pen over—where the zebras were. It knew.

Fast forward a couple decades, I was barely functional when my Helen drove me sixty miles each week, through driving rain, winter snow, and deepest dark to a Peer-to-Peer class offered by the National Alliance on Mental Illness (NAMI). Peer-to-Peer goes largely in the education category, but the support it offered as well was incalculable. The classes are for all kinds of wonky brains, and the two dozen of us ran the gamut. After a couple weeks spent sitting around a large rectangle of tables, I noticed a pattern. Mood disorders sat to the right, OCD and borderline to the left. People with schizoaffective and schizophrenia took up the middle, edging over to the bipolar side as the weeks went by. Were we less scary than the cutters? Did they recognize us as fellow travelers in more imaginative lands? In any case, we knew. Not separated by fences, we found our kin.

These people did not become my bosom buddies. They lived sixty miles away. But for two hours a week, not to be the one who was different . . .

Sometimes I learn a lot from my peers in support groups, sometimes I find help with my issue, sometimes not. But for that hour or two, I can exhale.

Other people help too. Bipolar is not a DIY project. Doctors and therapists, friends and family can drive you nuts. They can also keep you from going too nuts. These people are your early warning system when your own warning system fails. The doc who said, "I notice your thoughts are not as organized as they usually are . . ." My wife who says, "Your voice is getting louder . . ." Can I dial it back, draw on my bag of self-care tricks? If not, it's time to get help from somebody else.

It's a tricky business. You are the one who knows what it's like in your skin. You are the one who knows best what your values are. But some days your brain is held hostage, and you are not in the best position to make decisions about how to get to the life you want to live.

There are certain kinds of help I do not want. In the past I have hidden my symptoms to prevent receiving unwanted help. The danger with that strategy is that the farther out on the edge one travels without a steadying hand, the greater the chance for the hard fall.

A plan, work out a plan, this time a different kind of plan. My therapist and I, my wife and I talk about early warning signals. We negotiate what will happen when the signals show up.

Many states have psychiatric advance directives, where you can detail the kind of treatment you want to receive or not receive while in the hospital. I don't know if they work, even assuming the docs know about your advance directives. Options for care are limited these days. And ultimately, the docs have the legal obligation to do what they think they need to do. But an advance directive can give them a heads-up on how this particular patient might respond to that particular treatment and, where there are options, to choose the one that will work best.

The plans short of hospitalization are more sure. I'm talking simple things, like, if my wife thinks I am edging out of control, even if I don't, I agree to call my therapist.

Then I do my best to tell them and tell myself the truth.

Medication

In 2012 when I moved to Central Oregon, all the local psychiatrists rejected patients on either Medicare or disability. Sigh. It turned out OK, because with the help of a doc who reads my blog, I got in to see the man who would turn out to be my fourth psychiatrist, The Expert. He is on the other side of the Cascades, it's a two-hour drive, and the roads close in winter. But I'm usually stable now, and he is worth the drive. He wrote the book, a couple books, on the bipolar spectrum. He told me, "You are in the driver's seat. Your family physician is sitting next to you. I'll be in the back seat, making suggestions."

With an attitude like that, I was willing to listen.

I couldn't tolerate the side effects of the first mood stabilizer he suggested. We were discussing his second choice, about which I was dubious, when he said, "I think you may be one of those people who is opposed to taking medication."

I looked at him. I thought, *I know where you got that in your book,* but what I said was, "I don't know where you got that in my chart"—which had twenty psych meds in my history at this point.

Point to me.

I continued, "I am concerned about trying this new one because I have had bad reactions to so many in the past."

"You had bad reactions because you were taking the wrong meds."

Point to him.

And the Chemistry Experiment continued, though this time with a higher level of trust, because The Expert knows that patients won't take meds that make us feel worse. He even tells other psychiatrists this news flash—their patients won't take meds that make them feel worse. He often recommends lower doses and a heavy reliance on all the other recovery strategies I have been describing.

Remember Sarah Russell's study of one hundred people with bipolar who are symptom-free or in control of their condition? Eighty-five percent of them are on meds, which they adjust for microscopic shifts in mood and energy. Many combine Western-style meds with alternative treatments.

Meds are lower on the list of strategies to maintain recovery, though depending on where you are on the spectrum, they may still be a daily requirement. Meds move to the top of the list in a crisis. Most people can decrease their dose once they've come down off the ceiling. Lower doses often decrease side effects, which increases the likelihood you will keep taking them if you get a benefit from them. Talk to your doc.

I have a friend whose last manic episode destroyed her marriage, her bank account, her relationship with her kids, her life. She wants high doses. She would rather live partially numbed than ever risk a repeat performance.

Me, I have never quite experienced those ravages. Misdiagnosis and the wrong treatment ended my career. But my danger has been primarily to myself. I have tried every mood stabilizer on the shelf, and way too much of the antidepressant shelf, with the goal of improving my life. I will try almost anything. But if I can't function on it, I won't take it.

This is called weighing your costs and benefits. For my friend, the cost of mania is higher than the benefit of a clear head. For me, full-blown mania is remote, while being able to write is what gets me out of bed in the morning. Hospitalization would change the calculation. Yes, I will take an antipsychotic if I am psychotic. But I won't do it to tweak what has been working for five years now.

If you are on meds or your doctor thinks you should be, take note: I said you might be able to decrease your dose, not quit. When something is working, when you are finally feeling good, why on God's good earth would you quit? Medication is one of the tools in the recovery toolbox. A philosophical objection to medication makes no more sense than a philosophical objection to screwdrivers.

Still, medication is just one tool. You need more tools than a screwdriver if you're going to fix that collapsed roof.

The Recovery Model

The steps to recovery are crisis, rebuilding, and transformation.

In a *crisis*, when symptoms flare and leave us unable to take responsibility for ourselves, we need people to take care of us, to provide safety and medication, and then recuperation, shelter, sleep, and food.

After the crisis, we *rebuild* our sense of self. We need to tell our story, have others hear our pain, and learn about what is happening to us. Others can encourage us and offer practical help. This is where peers, therapy, and learning skills come in.

When we have come through the fire, we don't get our old life back. But we are not just "the person with the mental illness" either. We are *transformed*. We begin to dream again about who we can be. This is the stage of self-acceptance, confidence, assertiveness, helping others, building a different life but a life still worth living.

Too often there is a mismatch between stage and intervention. They pile on the education during a three-day hospital stay when you are too doped up to take it in. Then they insist on continuing levels of medication that preclude ever leaving the house except to get your refills, until you are so bored you go off your meds entirely, if only for something different.

If somebody has told you to just take your meds for the rest of your life and your life will be normal, that person has lied to you and deserves to rot in hell for exposing you to disaster. Instead, take responsibility for your health. Pay attention to what is happening, figure out what intervention you need, and go get it.

It's not a straight-line process, ever upward. Bipolar is a remitting, recurring condition, like the game Chutes and Ladders. Relapse is part of this picture. If you take care of yourself, you don't have to slide as often or as far. But you may still slide.

Dammit.

When relapse happens, figure out your current stage, then get and accept the help needed at that stage. The sooner you do, the sooner you will be on your way again.

If I could go back a decade and send a text to my sorry soul, which could no longer deny the diagnosis I did not want to have, it would say:

Go ahead and grieve. You have lost a lot and soon will lose more. But it will get better. It will. Learn what you need to learn. Do what you need to do. Now you have a shot.

Choose life.

A Voice from the Edge

Keep Going—Resources

The more you know, the more tools you have to get better. This is a sampling of what I have found helpful. Start anywhere, start with whatever catches your interest.

Diagnosis and Treatment

MDQ and BSDS: These diagnostic instruments are in the appendix following this chapter. There is a third screening tool called MoodCheck, combining symptoms with other markers of life experience that influence the likelihood of the disorder. You can find it and a whole lot of information about diagnosis and treatment at PsychEducation.org.

Online: NAMI.org (the National Alliance on Mental Illness) is your one-stop shop for education, support, and advocacy. Under the About Mental Illness tab, there is a list of all kinds of mental illnesses with more information as you dive into the links.

Book: Chris Aiken and James Phelps, *Bipolar, Not So Much: Understanding Your Mood Swings and Depression.* This is the next book to read. Phelps and Aiken explain the bipolar spectrum for a popular audience, recommend a number of self-help strategies, describing them in detail, list the pros and cons of the various medical treatments, and discuss recovery.

Recovery

Face-to-face: NAMI's signature Peer-to-Peer is a free, eight-session educational program for people who are ready to get going on their recovery. Peer-to-Peer is taught by people who have been there and are still on the journey. It offers information, tools, support, and hope. Find more at nami.org/peertopeer.

Face-to-face: Back to NAMI for the NAMI Connection Recovery Support Group. This is not another group of unhappy people sitting around to vent. The group is led by trained facilitators who are also living with a mental illness to help us learn from each other. This site will help you find a local meeting: nami.org/connection.

Book: Ellen Frank, *Treating Bipolar Disorder: A Clinician's Guide to Interpersonal and Social Rhythm Therapy*. Frank did not write this book for you, the one in the pajamas. She wrote it for your therapist. Look past the stigmatizing language that seems inevitable when clinicians talk with each other. She is less stigmatizing than most. If you find an IPSRT-trained therapist, it will be by luck. There are not a lot of them, and while they have a website designed for clinicians, there still seems to be no referral point for patients to find therapists. But you can work the social rhythms part out on your own and ask your therapist to help with the interpersonal part. Search online for briefer introductions to IPSRT.

Humor

Seriously, there is a lot out there. Search online for bipolar humor, depression humor, suicide humor. Yes, suicide humor. The following are two of my favorites.

Podcast: *The Hilarious World of Depression* is brought to you by makeitok.org and features John Moe interviewing comedians who have depression, many of whom have YouTubes of their performances and websites of their own. Visit hilariousworld.org.

Comic Book: *Hyperbole and a Half*, by Allie Brosh, is a graphic novel about depression and anxiety.

Its partner, hyperboleandahalf.blogspot.com, is a blog.

Zebras (finding people like you)

Face-to-face: See NAMI's Peer-to-Peer and Connection Recovery Groups on the previous page to find fellow travelers.

Face-to-face and online: Depression and Bipolar Support Alliance is a smaller version of NAMI. The most significant difference between the two is that DBSA is by and for the people who have mood disorders themselves, while NAMI was founded by parents of people with schizophrenia. NAMI's mission has expanded to include education and advocacy about all mental illnesses and people who have them, but peers, those with the illness, still struggle to find a voice in some chapters. NAMI is trying to change this dynamic. They are making progress. But that's the difference. Caveat: I have not attended DBSA meetings myself. The closest for me is on the other side of those mountains. They also have online support groups: dbsalliance.org.

Online forums: Honestly, use these with caution. You can read descriptions of the disasters that ensued when somebody took some particular medication and be reassured you are not the only one. You can vent about your own anxieties and disasters. You can learn tips for handling side effects. But do not get your medical advice from them. Do. Not. They are as reliable as the latest scandal your Facebook friend did not fact-check. Do not ever quote something from them to your doctor. Do. Not.

Blogs: Blogs come and go. I am reluctant to recommend specific ones. Well, there's mine, of course, prozacmonologues.com. Try searching *best bipolar blogs* or something similar and consider the source of the list. There are other good ones out there.

For Friends and Family
Face-to-face: Again from NAMI, Family-to-Family. This eight-session course offers education and support for family and friends. Find it at nami.org/find-support/nami-programs/nami-family-to-family.

Book: David L. Conroy, *Out of the Nightmare: Recovery from Depression and Suicidal Pain.* Best thing I have ever read on this subject. Conroy makes sense of why suicide happens and gives advice for how to prevent it. "Suicide is not a choice; it happens when pain exceeds resources for coping with pain." The book is written for those who suffer, for friends and family, and for society.

Book: Sheila Hamilton, *All the Things We Never Knew: Chasing the Chaos of Mental Illness.* Hamilton's heartbreaking memoir of her husband's suicide demonstrates the nightmare of ignorance and isolation. Her story did not have to go this way. Reach out. Contact NAMI.

For Clinicians
Book: James Phelps, *A Spectrum Approach to Mood Disorders: Not Fully Bipolar But Not Unipolar—Practical Management.* Phelps wrote this book specifically for clinicians, going beyond DSM checklists to acknowledge the more complicated lived experience of patients. Addressing the concept of the mood spectrum, differential diagnosis, real-world scenarios, treatment guidelines, nonmedical approaches, as well as the usual bipolar medications and other treatments, Phelps offers a comprehensive guide for

professionals who treat people who inhabit the broad territory between classic expressions of major depression and Bipolar I, the spectrum.

Book: Ellen Frank, *Treating Bipolar Disorder: A Clinician's Guide to Interpersonal and Social Rhythm Therapy.* Frank's book is also written for clinicians, a thorough description of the theory and practice of IPSRT. Her department now offers online training at ipsrt.org.

Brain Stuff
Coloring Book: Marian C. Diamond and Arnold B. Scheibel, *The Human Brain Coloring Book* is designed for students in psychology or medicine or anyone who wants to learn about the brain. You learn as you color plates that illustrate brain structures, neurons, calcium channels, brain development, and more. There are a number of coloring books out there. I like this one.

Online: Neuroscientifically Challenged is a website with articles, two-minute videos, a glossary, and lots of diagrams. It is a handy place to go when you are reading about the brain and come across a term you don't know. Or it can be where you learn more about the brain one bit at a time: neuroscientificallychallenged.com. The author, Mark Kingman, also has a book, *Your Brain Explained.*

Book: Frederick Goodwin and Kay Redfield Jamison, *Manic-Depressive Illness: Bipolar Disorders and Recurrent Depression* is the challenge book, 976 pages of everything scientists know about manic-depressive illness, with the benefit that one of these scientists has Bipolar I herself and the other knows her as a professional first, not as an odd specimen with a few redeeming features that fail to compensate for the problems she causes her associates when she decides there is a snake outbreak in Los Angeles, and she has to stock the city with snakebite kits . . . The book was first published in 1990, revised in 2007. But it still covers the territory.

Goodwin and Jamison lay out the historical and, they assert, more correct paradigm of bipolar, that the essential feature is not mood but rather cycling. They prefer the older name, note the title, rather than the confusing *bipolar*, which directs you to the single feature of up and down. Hence, they belong in the bipolar spectrum camp. You could call them the senior camp counselors of the bipolar spectrum camp.

Manic-Depressive Illness is for people who want to dig into the textbook aspiring psychiatrists read. Sections include clinical description and diagnosis, clinical studies, psychological studies, pathophysiology, and treatment. They cover everything from DNA sites to cellular plasticity to sleep to creativity. You don't need to know all this stuff, unless you are an aspiring psychiatrist. Like, I skimmed the chapter on signaling networks and calcium channels. Use the table of contents to find your way to the comprehensible parts.

Book: John McManamy, *Not Just Up and Down.* The DSM is the linear thinker's paradise. The reality it purports to describe is messy. Everything is interconnected. By everything, McManamy means symptoms, life experiences, personality traits, and daily habits. What if we could tear up the DSM and start over? This time listen to patients and use their experiences to create a new classification for mental disorders. Somebody has to do it, reasons McManamy. Why not him?

McManamy is reaching farther than the NIMH and Insel for his data. He is what you call an expert patient. He has done his homework. He has street cred with psychiatrists. Well, he has on occasion been invited to present at their conferences, until he tells them something they don't want to hear. He is also a funny guy.

Not Just Up and Down is the first of a series that continues with *In Search of Identity* and *Arriving: Principles in Recovery.*

From God to Neurons

The following have a bit of everything.

Online: *You Are Your Own Expert: McMan's Depression and Bipolar Web* is a huge resource center designed to help you learn what you want to learn: mcmanweb.com.

Online: *Prozac Monologues: Reflections and Research on the Mind, the Brain, Mental Illness, and Society* is what I do when I am not writing a book. You'll find articles, videos, rants, a sermon or two, and links to other resources: prozacmonologues.com.

Magazine, paper, and online: The website bphope.com is affiliated with *bp Magazine* and has articles about the latest research, treatment, relationships, personal stories, tips, inspiration, and blogs. You can get a paper copy too.

The learning, the recovery, the rest of your life has begun. It will be worth it. It will. Keep going.

APPENDIX

Mood Disorder Questionnaire (MDQ)

Reprinted from *American Journal of Psychiatry*, Vol 157, No. 11, Robert M. A. Hirschfeld, Janet B. W. Williams, Robert L. Spitzer, Joseph R. Calabrese, Laurie Flynn, Paul E. Keck, Lydia Lewis, Susan L. McElroy, and Robert M. Post. "Development and Validation of a Screening Instrument for Bipolar Spectrum Disorder: The Mood Disorder Questionnaire," 1873–75. Copyright 2000, with permission by RMA Hirschfeld, MD.

1. Has there ever been a time in your life when you were not your usual self and . . .

   . . . you felt so good or so hyper that other people thought you were not your normal self or you were so hyper that you got into trouble?

   . . . you were so irritable that you shouted at people or started fights or arguments?

   . . . you felt much more self-confident than usual?

   . . . you got much less sleep than usual and found you didn't really miss it?

   . . . you were much more talkative or spoke much faster than usual?

   . . . thoughts raced through your head or you couldn't slow your mind down?

. . . you were so easily distracted by things around you that you had trouble concentrating or staying on track?

. . . you had much more energy than usual?

. . . you were much more active or did many more things than usual?

. . . you were much more social or outgoing than usual, for example, you telephoned friends in the middle of the night?

. . . you were much more interested in sex than usual?

. . . you did things that were unusual for you or that other people might have thought were excessive, foolish, or risky?

. . . spending money got you or your family in trouble?

2. If you have checked YES to more than one of the above, have several of these ever happened during the same period of time?

3. How much of a problem did any of these cause you—like being unable to work; having family, money or legal troubles; getting into arguments or fights? Please circle one response only.

- No problem
- Minor problem
- Moderate problem
- Serious problem

4. Have any of your blood relatives (i.e. children, siblings, parents, grandparents, aunts, uncles) had manic-depressive illness or bipolar disorder?

5. Has a health professional ever told you that you have manic-depressive illness or bipolar disorder?

If you answer:

1. "Yes" to seven or more of the 13 items in question number 1; AND
2. "Yes" to the co-occurrence item (question number 2); AND
3. "Moderate" or "Serious" to question number 3 (degree of functional impairment) then you have a positive screen. All three of the criteria above should be met. A positive screen should be followed by a comprehensive medical evaluation for Bipolar Spectrum Disorder.

Bipolar Spectrum Diagnostic Scale

Reprinted from *Journal of Affective Disorders*, Vol 84, No. 2–3, S. Nassir Ghaemi, Christopher Miller, Douglas Berv, Jeffry Klugman, Klara J. Rosenquist, and Ronald W. Pies. "Sensitivity and Specificity of a New Bipolar Spectrum Diagnostic Scale," 273–77. Copyright 2005, with permission from Elsevier.

Instructions:

1. Please read through the entire passage below before filling in any blanks.

Some individuals notice that their mood and/or energy levels shift drastically from time to time___. These individuals notice that, at times, their mood and/or energy level is very low, and at other times, very high___. During their "low" phases, these individuals often feel a lack of energy; a need to stay in bed or get extra sleep; and little or no motivation to do things they need to do___. They often put on weight during these periods___. During their low phases, these individuals often feel "blue", sad all the time, or depressed___. Sometimes, during these low phases, they feel hopeless or even suicidal___. Their ability to function at work or socially is impaired___. Typically, these low phases last for a few weeks, but sometimes they last only a few days___. Individuals with this type of pattern may experience a period of "normal" mood in between mood swings, during which their mood and energy level feels "right" and their ability to function is not disturbed___. They may then notice a marked shift or "switch" in the way they feel___. Their energy increases above what is normal for them, and they often get many things done they would not ordinarily be able to do___. Sometimes, during these "high" periods, these individuals feel as if they have too much energy or feel "hyper"___. Some individuals, during these high periods, may feel irritable, "on edge", or aggressive___. Some individuals, during these high periods, take on too many activities at once___. During these high periods, some individuals may spend money in ways that cause them trouble___. They may be more talkative, outgoing, or sexual during these periods___. Sometimes, their behavior during these high periods seems strange or annoying to others___. Sometimes, these individuals get into difficulty with coworkers or the police, during these high periods___. Sometimes, they increase their alcohol or non-prescription drug use during these high periods___.

2. Now that you have read this passage, please check one of the following four boxes:

- ❑ This story fits me very well, or almost perfectly
- ❑ This story fits me fairly well
- ❑ This story fits me to some degree but not in most respects
- ❑ This story does not really describe me at all

3. Now please go back and put a check after each sentence that definitely describes you.

BSDS Scoring:

Each sentence checked is worth one point. Add six points for "fits me very well," four points for "fits me fairly well," and two points for "fits me to some degree."

Total score likelihood of bipolar disorder:

0–6 Highly unlikely
7–12 Low risk
13–19 Moderate risk
20–25 High risk

Optimum threshold for positive diagnosis: score of 13 or above.

NOTES

Bizarre

1. **Twenty percent of the population of the United States will experience an episode of depression sometime over their lifetimes:** Hasin, "Epidemiology of Adult DSM-5 Major Depressive Disorder and Its Specifiers in the United States." These numbers are rising. The original text has been updated to reflect figures from 2018.

2. **Half of them a whole lot of episodes:** Kessler, "The Epidemiology of Depression across Cultures." More than two episodes is called *recurrent depression.*

3. **Half are sometimes way up, but more often way down:** Benazzi, "Bipolar II Disorder: Current Issues in Diagnosis and Management." Benazzi examined how many of all people with depression experience symptoms of hypomania or mania, whether or not they meet the full diagnostic criteria for bipolar.

4. **Another 1.5 percent feel lousy all the time:** National Institute of Mental Health, "Persistent Depressive Disorder (Dysthymic Disorder)." According to NIMH, persistent depressive disorder, also known as dysthymic disorder, is low-level depression that persists for two years or longer.

Jump

1. Sixty-three percent of the people who attempt suicide do so while experiencing a mixed episode: Balázs, "The Close Link between Suicide Attempts and Mixed (Bipolar) Depression: Implications for Suicide Prevention." In this sample, 70.8 percent of suicide attempters who were depressed had three or more symptoms of hypomania. While people diagnosed with Bipolar II were already overrepresented among the suicide attempters, the authors believe that even more may have been overlooked because the current diagnostic system fails to identify them.

Making the Call

1. Bipolar disorder is not diagnosed . . . for an average of 7.5 years: Singh, "Misdiagnosis of Bipolar Disorder." These rates are not improving over time.

2. Irritability and psychomotor agitation are the strongest predictors of the jump: Balázs, "The Close Link between Suicide Attempts and Mixed (Bipolar) Depression." The authors recommend that every case of depression should be assessed for mixed features.

3. Half the people in the unipolar drawer eventually get switched to the bipolar drawer: "Across the entire lifetime, every new episode of depression brings a new risk for mania," one study concludes. This finding supports the theory that recurrent depression is more like bipolar than like single episode unipolar depression. Angst, "Diagnostic Conversion from Depression to Bipolar Disorders: Results of a Long-Term Prospective Study of Hospital Admissions."

4. Between 25 and 60 percent of persons with either Bipolar I or II attempt suicide at some time in their lives: Novick, "Suicide

Attempts in Bipolar I and Bipolar II Disorder: A Review and Meta-Analysis of The Evidence."

5. **The bipolar spectrum:** Cassano, "The Mood Spectrum in Unipolar and Bipolar Disorder: Arguments for a Unitary Approach." Simply expressed, the bipolar spectrum refers to the vast and varied area between a single episode of depression and the classic expression of Bipolar I. Kupfer was a co-author of this article from 2004.

6. **Lithium has the strongest record of success, though it works best for those who have the most classic version of Bipolar I:** Severus, "Lithium for Prevention Of Mood Episodes in Bipolar Disorders: Systematic Review and Meta-Analysis." Lithium leads the list for prevention of mania. It is not the first choice for prevention of depression. Since depression is harder to treat and since it follows hard upon an episode of mania, a common strategy is to focus on preventing the mania.

7. **Mixed episodes:** Muneer, "Mixed States in Bipolar Disorder: Etiology, Pathogenesis and Treatment." The DSM-5 now recognizes the significance of episodes that combine manic and depressive symptoms, which pose particular dangers and complications for treatment.

8. **The experts call this antidepressant-plus-mood-stabilizer approach controversial:** Ghaemi, "Treatment of Rapid-Cycling Bipolar Disorder: Are Antidepressants Mood Destabilizers?" There are two issues here. Some doctors prescribe mood stabilizers along with antidepressants thinking to avoid the "switch," a manic episode provoked by the antidepressant alone. The Systematic Treatment Enhancement Program for Bipolar Disorder (STEP-BD) demonstrated that this approach results in rapid cycling, or more frequent episodes. Indeed, rapid cycling simply was not described by clinicians until the 1970s, after antidepressants began to be used.

9. **Antidepressants and suicide:** Rihmer, "Suicide Risk in Mood Disorders." The suicide/antidepressant link appears to be mediated by mixed episodes, when antidepressants provoke manic/hypomanic symptoms in people with unidentified bipolarity. See the earlier discussion of Cymbalta.

10. **Antidepressants and suicide:** Rihmer, "Do Antidepressants T(h)reat(en) Depressives? Toward a Clinically Judicious Formulation of the Antidepressant-Suicidality FDA Advisory in Light of Declining National Suicide Statistics from Many Countries." Antidepressants do seem to prevent suicide in seriously depressed people. When those who should not be taking them (because of unidentified bipolarity) are removed from the sample, the authors believe the statistics for their success would be more robust.

11. **Antidepressants and suicide:** Berk, "Are Treatment Emergent Suicidality and Decreased Response to Antidepressants in Younger Patients Due to Bipolar Disorder Being Misdiagnosed as Unipolar Depression?" Younger patients are at particular risk, since so many doctors believe that children and adolescents do not have bipolar disorder. The diagnosis (with its appropriate medication) is not considered until after disaster strikes in one form or another.

Three

1. **The memory impairments of depression:** Kihlstrom, "Emotion and Memory: Implications for Self-Report." Everybody, not just those who have a mental illness, finds it easier to remember events that are "mood congruent." When depressed, it is easier to remember sad things. When happy, we more easily remember happy things.

2. **Only 22 percent of those with a previous . . . episode even recognized it:** "Respondents [in the study] gave alternative

explanations for their manic symptoms, explaining them as pleasant and productive periods, part of their personality, and as a result of various psychosocial circumstances." That is for "happy" hypomania. If the symptoms combine with a depressive episode, they are simply taken to be part of the depression by patients and too often doctors alike. Regeer, "Low Self-Recognition and Awareness of Past Hypomanic and Manic Episodes in the General Population."

3. **Your score tells you how likely it is you really do need to check this out further:** Ghaemi, "Sensitivity and Specificity of a New Bipolar Spectrum Diagnostic Scale." The instrument detects 75 percent of those with Bipolar I and 79 percent of those with Bipolar II, with a "false positive" of 15 percent for those with unipolar depression.

4. **Akiskal . . . has his own approach, called "The Rule of Three":** Akiskal, "Searching for Behavioral Indicators of Bipolar II in Patients Presenting with Major Depressive Episodes: The 'Red Sign,' the 'Rule Of Three' and Other Biographic Signs of Temperamental Extravagance, Activation and Hypomania." Akiskal's work shows that the "softer" end of the bipolar spectrum is more likely to reveal itself through "behavioral activation" (excess activity) than elevated mood. One reason doctors miss this diagnosis is because the Structured Clinical Interview for DSM (SCID) begins its exploration of the bipolar possibility with a question about mood and excludes the diagnosis if the patient doesn't remember or acknowledge elevated mood.

Metaphor

1. **DepressionHurts.com:** Alas, the website I described in 2007 has been taken down.

2. **Lands' End:** This feature is no longer available at the Lands' End website. Now, its loss really is a tragedy; it was wonderfully helpful and fun.

3. **The history of the Chemistry Experiment:** Barondes, "Fresh Air."

Balancing Act

1. **Anxiety could be considered a key feature of some variants of the condition:** Sagman, "Comorbidity in Bipolar Disorder." Bipolar is something of an umbrella term that covers a range of similar conditions. Half of those with bipolar disorder also have anxiety. The two may sit side by side as comorbid conditions. Or there may be an underlying mechanism common to both, so that for some, anxiety is part of how their bipolar manifests.

2. **Brain nerds can describe it in one paragraph:** Maletic, "Integrated Neurobiology of Bipolar Disorder." Maletic has diagrammed this developmental process in an elegant illustration of interacting factors.

3. **To maintain homeostasis:** Goodwin and Jamison, *Manic-Depressive Illness: Bipolar Disorders and Recurrent Depression,* 599.

4. **A whole series of mistimings and misalignments in our internal and external cycles results in a failure to rebalance:** Maletic, "Integrated Neurobiology of Bipolar Disorder." An examination of what is happening inside the brain reveals enormous complexity across many functions and systems. Many of these mistimings and misalignments are operating even in the absence of mood symptoms. It's not just up and down!

5. **People with bipolar have a flattened cortisol curve:** Havermans, "Patterns of Salivary Cortisol Secretion and Responses to Daily

Events in Patients with Remitted Bipolar Disorder." The more episodes a patient has, the higher the cortisol level overall and the flatter the curve, even when in remission.

6. **Little critters inside our cells called mitochondria:** Konradi, "Molecular Evidence for Mitochondrial Dysfunction in Bipolar Disorder." Konradi's team found dysregulation of energy metabolism particularly in the hippocampus, the source of memory. On a more popular level, Madeleine L'Engle's children's science fiction book *A Wind in the Door* has a plot that revolves around the centrality of mitochondria in energy production.

7. **There was a gap between the part of my brain that knew I had done everything . . . and the part of my brain that was on full red-alarm alert:** The automatic/internal network modulates feeling states that arise from within, e.g., in response to memories. The volitional/external network handles emotional states in response to external events. "These two networks have shared components and collaboratively regulate amygdala responses in complex emotional circumstances." That's the way it is supposed to work, anyway! Maletic, "Integrated Neurobiology of Bipolar Disorder."

8. **The more manic episodes you have, the bigger these holes:** Strakowski, "Ventricular and Periventricular Structural Volumes in First- Versus Multiple-Episode Bipolar Disorder." This study compared the ventricles of people in their first episode of mania with those of people who had multiple episodes and healthy controls. The conclusions could be strengthened with a longitudinal study examining how each person's brain developed over time.

Wait, wait!

1. Insel, "Transforming Diagnosis."

2. **The brains of people who do better with medication are wired differently from the brains of those who do better with cognitive therapy:** McGrath, "Toward a Neuroimaging Treatment Selection Biomarker for Major Depressive Disorder." This study was funded by the NIMH and illustrates the significance of Insel's recommendation. Patients who are suffering currently waste time in blind experiments to find the treatment that will help and bear the physical and financial costs of treatments that do not help.

3. **In one experiment, identifying faces with neutral expressions and faces expressing disgust:** Lagopoulos, "Impairments in 'Top-Down' Processing in Bipolar Disorder: A Simultaneous fMRI–GSR Study." Both groups could distinguish the faces accurately. But the results point to the difficulty that people with bipolar have in evaluating the significance of emotional stimuli because the reacting part of the brain engages before the thinking part.

4. **Similar experiments have distinguished between people with bipolar and people with major depression . . . while in remission:** Han, "Differentiating between Bipolar and Unipolar Depression in Functional and Structural MRI Studies." This article is a review of literature. There are lots of studies examining the differences between how the brains of people with bipolar and people with major depression function differently (sometimes with contradictory findings).

5. **Similar experiments have distinguished between people with bipolar and people with major depression . . . during a depressive episode:** Fateh, "Hippocampal Functional Connectivity-Based Discrimination between Bipolar and Major Depressive Disorders." Being able to tell the difference between bipolar depression

and major depression during a depressive episode would have the greatest clinical significance, since this is the point at which people are first diagnosed.

6. **Yet another experiment used fMRI and a spatial working memory test . . . particularly useful when diagnosing children with behavior difficulties:** Brauser, "fMRI Distinguishes between Bipolar Disorder and ADHD." It is believed that bipolar is rare in children, leading doctors to not consider the diagnosis and reinforcing the belief. The consequence of delayed treatment is a worse prognosis as time goes on.

7. **Bipolar overlaps more with schizophrenia than with major depression in cortical gene activity:** Dengler, "Major Mental Illnesses Unexpectedly Share Brain Gene Activity, Raising Hope for Better Diagnostics and Therapies." The cortical area, or cortex, is the thinking center of the brain. When the DSM conceives of schizophrenia primarily as a thought disorder and bipolar primarily as a mood disorder like depression, it obscures the cognitive dysfunctions in bipolar disorder. In truth, the cognitive symptoms of bipolar are frequently more disabling than the mood symptoms. People with bipolar might benefit from more research into this overlap with schizophrenia.

8. **Even EKGs . . . have been able to distinguish:** Hage, "Low Cardiac Vagal Tone Index by Heart Rate Variability Differentiates Bipolar from Major Depression." Here is an easy, non-invasive diagnostic tool already available.

9. **Even . . . blood levels of inflammation have been able to distinguish:** Brunoni, "Differences in the Immune-Inflammatory Profiles of Unipolar and Bipolar Depression."

Recovery

1. It screws up the GABA/glutamate balance: Wahls, *Minding My Mitochondria: How I Overcame Secondary Progressive Multiple Sclerosis (MS) and Got Out of My Wheelchair.* Wahls's book about MS addresses the effect of diet on a wide variety of chronic conditions, including mental illness. She gives detailed explanations of how the brain works to produce the energy it needs to function and how different foods support or hinder that process.

2. The stop and go hormones in your brain: Petroff, "GABA and Glutamate in the Human Brain." GABA and glutamate function in relation to each other. Petroff gives more detail about how this cycle works, including the role of glucose (a type of sugar).

3. Learning stimulates BDNF: Cunha, "A Simple Role for BDNF in Learning and Memory?" While a depletion of BDNF makes learning difficult, studies of rats have demonstrated that learning itself increases BDNF.

BIBLIOGRAPHY

Aiken, Chris. "Antidepressants in Bipolar II Disorder." *Psychiatric Times* 36, no. 5 (May 14, 2019). www.psychiatrictimes.com/bipolar-disorder/antidepressants-bipolar-ii-disorder.

———. "The Bipolar Spectrum: Practical Tips for Diagnosis and Treatment." *The Carlat Psychiatry Report* 16, no. 1 (January 2018): 1–5.

———. "The Secret Life of Bipolar Disorder." *Psychiatric Times* (March 7, 2017). www.psychiatrictimes.com/bipolar-disorder/secret-life-bipolar-disorder.

Aiken, Chris, and James Phelps. *Bipolar, Not So Much: Understanding Your Mood Swings and Depression.* New York: W.W. Norton & Company, 2017.

Akiskal, Hagop S. "The Emergence of the Bipolar Spectrum: Validation along Clinical-Epidemiologic and Familial-Genetic Lines." *Psychopharmacology Bulletin* 40, no. 4 (2007): 99–115.

———. "The Prevalent Clinical Spectrum of Bipolar Disorders: Beyond DSM-IV." *Journal of Clinical Psychopharmacology* 16, no. 2 suppl. 1 (April 1996): 4S–14S.

———. "Searching for Behavioral Indicators of Bipolar II in Patients Presenting with Major Depressive Episodes: The 'Red Sign,' the

'Rule of Three' and Other Biographic Signs of Temperamental Extravagance, Activation and Hypomania." *Journal of Affective Disorders* 84, no. 2–3 (February 2005): 279–90.

Akiskal, Hagop S., and Franco Benazzi. "Optimizing the Detection of Bipolar II Disorder in Outpatient Private Practice: Toward a Systematization of Clinical Diagnostic Wisdom." *Journal of Clinical Psychiatry* 66, no. 7 (July 2005): 914–21.

American Psychiatric Association. *Diagnostic and Statistical Manual of Mental Disorders, 5th ed.* Arlington, VA: American Psychiatric Publishing, 2013.

Amit, Ben H., and Abraham Weizman. "Antidepressant Treatment for Acute Bipolar Depression: An Update." *Depression Research and Treatment* (2012). http://dx.doi.org/10.1155/2012/684725.

Angst, Jules, Robert Sellaro, Hans H. Stassen, et al. "Diagnostic Conversion from Depression to Bipolar Disorders: Results of a Long-Term Prospective Study of Hospital Admissions." *Journal of Affective Disorders* 84, no. 2–3 (February 2005): 149–57.

Balázs, Judit, Franco Benazzi, Zoltán Rihmer, et al. "The Close Link between Suicide Attempts and Mixed (Bipolar) Depression: Implications for Suicide Prevention." *Journal of Affective Disorders* 91, no. 2-3 (2006): 133–38.

Baldessarini, Ross J., Leonardo Tondo, and John Hennen. "Treatment Delays in Bipolar Disorders." *American Journal of Psychiatry* 156, no. 5 (May 1999): 811–12.

Barondes, Samuel. Interview by Terry Gross, *Fresh Air*, National Public Radio, June 23, 2003.

Benazzi, Franco. "Bipolar II Disorder: Current Issues in Diagnosis and Management." *Psychiatric Times* 23, no. 9 (August 1, 2006). www.psychiatrictimes.com/bipolar-disorder/bipolar-ii-disorder-current-issues-diagnosis-and-management.

Berk, Michael, and Seetal Dodd. "Are Treatment Emergent Suicidality and Decreased Response to Antidepressants in Younger Patients Due to Bipolar Disorder Being Misdiagnosed as Unipolar Depression?" *Medical Hypotheses* 65, no. 1 (2005): 39–43.

Blumberg, Hilary P., Hoi-Chung Leung, Pawel Skudlarski, et al. "A Functional Magnetic Resonance Imaging Study of Bipolar Disorder: State- and Trait-Related Dysfunction in Ventral Prefrontal Cortices." *Archives of General Psychiatry* 60, no. 6 (June 2003): 601–09.

Brauser, Deborah. "fMRI Distinguishes Between Bipolar Disorder and ADHD." *Medscape Medical News* (June 16, 2011). www.medscape.com/viewarticle/744742.

Brosh, Allie. *Hyperbole and a Half: Unfortunate Situations, Flawed Coping Mechanisms, Mayhem, and Other Things That Happened.* New York, NY: Touchstone Books, 2013.

Brunoni, Andre R., Thitiporn Supasitthumrong, Antonio Lucio Teixeira, et al. "Differences in the Immune-Inflammatory Profiles of Unipolar and Bipolar Depression." *Journal of Affective Disorders* 262 (February 2020): 8–15.

Carroll, B. J. "Clinical Science and Biomarkers: Against RDoC." *Acta Psychiatrica Scandinavica* 132, no. 6 (September 2015): 423–24.

Cassano, Giovanni B., Paola Rucci, Ellen Frank, David J. Kupfer, et al. "The Mood Spectrum in Unipolar and Bipolar Disorder: Arguments for a Unitary Approach." *American Journal of Psychiatry* 161, no. 7 (July 2004): 1264–69.

Conroy, David L. *Out of the Nightmare: Recovery from Depression and Suicidal Pain*. Lincoln, NE: Authors Choice Press, 2006.

Cunha, Carla, Riccardo Brambilla, and Kerrie L. Thomas. "A Simple Role for BDNF in Learning and Memory?" *Frontiers in Molecular Neuroscience* 3, no. 1 (February 2010).

Daban, C., E. Vieta, P. Mackin, and A. H. Young. "Hypothalamic-pituitary-adrenal Axis and Bipolar Disorder." *Psychiatric Clinics of North America* 28, no. 2 (June 2005): 469–80.

Dengler, Roni. "Major Mental Illnesses Unexpectedly Share Brain Gene Activity, Raising Hope for Better Diagnostics and Therapies." *Science Magazine* (February 8, 2018). www.sciencemag.org/news/2018/02/major-mental-illnesses-unexpectedly-share-brain-gene-activity-raising-hope-better.

Diamond, Marian C., and Arnold B. Scheibel. *The Human Brain Coloring Book (Coloring Concepts)*. New York: Collins Reference, 1985.

Eli Lilly and Company. "Highlights of Prescribing Information for Cymbalta." Updated October 2019. http://pi.lilly.com/us/cymbalta-pi.pdf.

Fateh, Ahmed Ameen, Zhiliang Long, Xujun Duan, et al. "Hippocampal Functional Connectivity-Based Discrimination between Bipolar and Major Depressive Disorders." *Psychiatry Research: Neuroimaging* 284 (February 2019): 53–60.

Frank, Ellen. *Treating Bipolar Disorder: A Clinician's Guide to Interpersonal and Social Rhythm Therapy.* New York: The Guilford Press, 2007.

Freeman, Marlene P., Scott Freeman, and Susan L. McElroy. "The Comorbidity of Bipolar and Anxiety Disorders: Prevalence, Psychobiology, and Treatment Issues." *Journal of Affective Disorders* 68, no. 1 (February 2002): 1–23.

Ghaemi, S. Nassir. "Treatment of Rapid-Cycling Bipolar Disorder: Are Antidepressants Mood Destabilizers?" *The American Journal of Psychiatry* 165, no. 3 (March 2008): 300–02.

Ghaemi, S. Nassir, Christopher Miller, Douglas Berv, et al. "Sensitivity and Specificity of a New Bipolar Spectrum Diagnostic Scale." *Journal of Affective Disorders* 84, no. 2–3 (February 2005): 273–77.

Goldberg, Joseph F., and Jessica L. Garno. "Development of Posttraumatic Stress Disorder in Adult Bipolar Patients with Histories of Severe Childhood Abuse." *Journal of Psychiatric Research* 39, no. 6 (November 2005): 595–601.

Goodfellow, Willa. *Prozac Monologues: Reflections and Research on the Mind, the Brain, Mental Illness, and Society.* www.prozacmonologues.com.

Goodwin, Frederick K., and Kay Redfield Jamison. *Manic-Depressive Illness: Bipolar Disorders and Recurrent Depression.* Oxford: Oxford University Press, 2007.

Grohol, John M. "Did the NIMH Withdraw Support for the DSM-5? No." *Psychcentral.com* (July 8, 2018). https://psychcentral.com/blog/did-the-nimh-withdraw-support-for-the-dsm-5-no/.

Hage, Brandon, Brianna Britton, David Daniels, et al. "Low Cardiac Vagal Tone Index by Heart Rate Variability Differentiates Bipolar from Major Depression." *World Journal of Biological Psychiatry* 20, no. 5 (2019): 359–67.

Hamilton, Sheila. *All the Things We Never Knew: Chasing the Chaos of Mental Illness.* New York: Seal Press, 2015.

Han, Kyu-Man, Domenico De Berardis, Michele Fornaro, et al. "Differentiating between Bipolar and Unipolar Depression in Functional and Structural MRI Studies." *Progress in Neuro-Psychopharmacology and Biological Psychiatry* 91 (April 2019): 20–27.

Hasin, Deborah S., Aaron L. Sarvet, Jacquelyn L. Meyers, et. al. "Epidemiology of Adult DSM-5 Major Depressive Disorder and Its Specifiers in the United States." *JAMA Psychiatry* 75, no. 4 (2018): 336–46.

Havermans, Rob, Nancy A. Nicolson, Johannes Berkhof, et al. "Patterns of Salivary Cortisol Secretion and Responses to Daily Events in Patients with Remitted Bipolar Disorder." *Psychoneuroendocrinology* 36, no. 2 (February 2011): 258–65.

Insel, Thomas. "Transforming Diagnosis." National Institute of Mental Health (April 29, 2013). www.nimh.nih.gov/about/directors/thomas-insel/blog/2013/transforming-diagnosis.shtml.

Kessler, Ronald C., and Evelyn J. Bromet. "The Epidemiology of Depression across Cultures." *Annual Review of Public Health* 34 (2013): 119–38.

Kihlstrom, John F., Eric Eich, Deborah Sandbrand, et al. "Emotion and Memory: Implications for Self-Report." In *The Science of*

Self-Report: Implications for Research and Practice, edited by Arthur A. Stone, Jaylan S. Turkkan, Christine A. Bachrach, et al. 81–99. Mahwah, NJ: Lawrence Erlbaum Associates Publishers, 2000.

Konradi, Christine, Molly Eaton, Matthew L. MacDonald, et al. "Molecular Evidence for Mitochondrial Dysfunction in Bipolar Disorder." *Archives of General Psychiatry* 61, no. 3 (March 2004): 300–08.

Korgaonkar, Mayuresh S., May Erlinger, Isabella A. Breukelaar, et al. "Amygdala Activation and Connectivity to Emotional Processing Distinguishes Asymptomatic Patients with Bipolar Disorders and Unipolar Depression." *Biological Psychiatry: Cognitive Neuroscience and Neuroimaging* 4, no. 4 (April 2019): 361–70.

Kushner, Harold S. *The Lord is My Shepherd: Healing Wisdom of the Twenty-third Psalm.* New York: Alfred A. Knopf, 2003.

Lagopoulos, Jim, and Gin Malhi. "Impairments In 'Top-Down' Processing in Bipolar Disorder: A Simultaneous fMRI–GSR Study." *Psychiatry Research: Neuroimaging* 192, no. 2 (May 2011): 100–08.

Lohano, Kavital, and Rif S. El-mallakh. "The Anxious Bipolar Patient." *Psychiatric Times* 28, no. 9 (September 6, 2011). www. psychiatrictimes.com/bipolar-disorder/anxious-bipolar-patient.

Maletic, Vladimir, and Charles Raison. "Integrated Neurobiology of Bipolar Disorder." *Frontiers in Psychiatry* 5, no. 98 (2014). https://doi.org/10.3389/fpsyt.2014.00098.

May, Gerald. *The Dark Night of the Soul: A Psychiatrist Explores the Connection Between Darkness and Spiritual Growth.* San Francisco: Harper San Francisco, 2004.

Mazure, Carolyn M., Gwendolyn P. Keita, and Mary C. Blehar. *Summit on Women and Depression: Proceedings and Recommendations.* Washington, DC: American Psychological Association, 2002.

McGrath, Callie L., Mary E. Kelley, Paul E. Holtzheimer III, et al. "Toward a Neuroimaging Treatment Selection Biomarker for Major Depressive Disorder." *JAMA Psychiatry* 70, no. 8 (June 12, 2013): 821-29. https://doi.org/10.1001/jamapsychiatry.2013.143.

Mcintyre, Roger S. "Novel Treatment Avenues for Bipolar Depression." *Psychiatric Times* 28, no. 4 (April 20, 2011). www.psychiatrictimes.com/bipolar-disorder/novel-treatment-avenues-bipolar-depression.

McManamy, John. *Not Just Up and Down: Understanding Mood in Bipolar Disorder.* John McManamy, 2015.

Meadows, Karen. *Searching for Normal: The Story of a Girl Gone Too Soon.* Berkeley: She Writes Press, 2016.

Moore, Thomas. *Dark Nights of the Soul: A Guide to Finding Your Way Through Life's Ordeals.* New York: Avery, 2005.

Muneer, Ather. "Mixed States in Bipolar Disorder: Etiology, Pathogenesis and Treatment." *Chonnam Medical Journal* 53, no. 1 (January 2017): 1–13.

Novick, Danielle M., Holly A. Swartz, and Ellen Frank. "Suicide Attempts in Bipolar I and Bipolar II Disorder: A Review and Meta-Analysis of the Evidence." *Bipolar Disorders* 12, no. 1 (February 2010): 1–9.

O'Donovan, Claire, Julie S. Garnham, Tomas Hajek, et al. "Antidepressant Monotherapy in Pre-Bipolar Depression: Predictive Value and Inherent Risk." *Journal of Affective Disorders* 107 (2008): 293–98.

Papolos, Demitri, and Janice Papolos. *Overcoming Depression: The Definitive Resource for Patients and Families Who Live with Depression and Manic-Depression*, 3rd ed. New York: HarperCollins, 1997.

Petroff, Ognen A.C. "GABA and Glutamate in the Human Brain." *Neuroscientist* 8, no. 6 (November 2002): 562–73.

Phelps, James. "Bipolar Disorder: The Year Ahead." *Psychiatric Times* (December 6, 2018). www.psychiatrictimes.com/bipolar-disorder/bipolar-disorder-year-ahead.

———. "A More Nuanced View of Hypomania." *Psychiatric Times* (February 7, 2017). www.psychiatrictimes.com/bipolar-disorder/more-nuanced-view-hypomania.

———. *A Spectrum Approach to Mood Disorders: Not Fully Bipolar But Not Unipolar—Practical Management*. New York: W. W. Norton & Company, 2016.

———. *Why Am I Still Depressed? Recognizing and Managing the Ups and Downs of Bipolar II and Soft Bipolar Disorder*. New York: McGraw Hill, 2006.

Pies, Ronald W. "Doctor, Is My Mood Disorder Due to a Chemical Imbalance?" *Psychiatric Times* (August 12, 2011). www.psychiatrictimes.com/couch-crisis/doctor-my-mood-disorder-due-chemical-imbalance.

———. "Is It Bipolar Depression? 'WHIPLASHED' Aids Diagnosis." *Current Psychiatry* 6, no. 3 (March 2007): 80–81.

Regeer, Eline J., Ralph W. Kupka, Margreet ten Have, et al. "Low Self-Recognition and Awareness of Past Hypomanic and Manic Episodes in the General Population." *International Journal of Bipolar Disorders* 3, no. 22 (2015). https://doi.org/10.1186/s40345-015-0039-8.

Rihmer, Zoltán. "Suicide Risk in Mood Disorders." *Current Opinion in Psychiatry* 20, no. 1 (2007): 17–22.

Rihmer, Zoltán, and Hagop S. Akiskal. "Do Antidepressants T(h)reat(en) Depressives? Toward a Clinically Judicious Formulation of the Antidepressant-Suicidality FDA Advisory in Light of Declining National Suicide Statistics from Many Countries." *Journal of Affective Disorders* 94, no. 1–3 (May 2006): 3–13.

Russell, Sarah. *A Lifelong Journey: Staying Well with Manic Depression/Bipolar Disorder.* Melbourne, Australia: Michelle Anderson Publishing, 2005.

Sagman, Doron, and Mauricio Tohen. "Comorbidity in Bipolar Disorder." *Psychiatric Times* 26, no. 4 (March 24, 2009). www.psychiatrictimes.com/bipolar-disorder/comorbidity-bipolar-disorder.

Saint John of the Cross. *Dark Night of the Soul.* Translated by Mirabai Starr. New York: Riverhead, 2003.

Schaffer, Charles B., Linda C. Schaffer, and Jeanne Howe. "Treatment-Resistant Bipolar Disorder." *Psychiatric Times* 34, no. 11 (November 27, 2017). www.psychiatrictimes.com/special-reports/treatment-resistant-bipolar-disorder-2017.

Severus, Emanuel, Matthew J. Taylor, Cathrin Sauer, et al. "Lithium for Prevention of Mood Episodes in Bipolar Disorders: Systematic Review and Meta-Analysis." *International Journal of Bipolar Disorders* 2, no. 15 (2014). https://doi.org/10.1186/s40345-014-0015-8.

Singh, Tanvir, and Muhammad Rajput. "Misdiagnosis of Bipolar Disorder." *Psychiatry (Edgmont)* 3, no. 10 (October 2006): 57–63.

Strakowski, Stephen M., Melissa P. DelBello, Molly E. Zimmerman, et al. "Ventricular and Periventricular Structural Volumes in First- Versus Multiple-Episode Bipolar Disorder." *The American Journal of Psychiatry* 159, no. 11 (November 2002): 1841–47.

Taber, Katherine H., Maurice Redden, and Robin A. Hurley. "Functional Anatomy of Humor: Positive Affect and Chronic Mental Illness." *The Journal of Neuropsychiatry and Clinical Neuroscience* 19, no. 4 (October 2007): 358–62.

U.S. Department of Health and Human Services. "Persistent Depressive Disorder (Dysthymic Disorder)." National Institute of Mental Health (November 2017). www.nimh.nih.gov/health/statistics/persistent-depressive-disorder-dysthymic-disorder.shtml.

U.S. Department of Health and Human Services. "Scan Predicts Whether Therapy or Meds Will Best Lift Depression."

National Institutes of Health (June 12, 2013). www.nih.gov/news-events/news-releases/scan-predicts-whether-therapy-or-meds-will-best-lift-depression.

Wahls, Terry. *Minding My Mitochondria: How I Overcame Secondary Progressive Multiple Sclerosis (MS) and Got Out of My Wheelchair.* Iowa City: TZ Press, 2010.

Wang, Chen, Karen Kerckhofs, Mark Van de Casteele, et al. "Glucose Inhibits GABA Release by Pancreatic Beta-Cells through an Increase in GABA Shunt Activity." *American Journal of Physiology: Endocrinology and Metabolism* 290, no. 3 (March 2006): E494–99.

ACKNOWLEDGMENTS

First there are the people who have simply (sometimes not so simply) helped to keep me on the planet: friends, colleagues, peers, therapists, doctors, musicians, authors, superheroes—how could I name you all? Know that I give thanks for you every day.

Then there are those who gave technical assistance: Dr. Ronald Pies, psychiatrist and ethicist at SUNY Upstate Medical University, Syracuse, NY, and Tufts University School of Medicine in Boston; and Dr. Jess Fiedorowicz, psychiatrist and researcher at Carver College of Medicine, University of Iowa, Iowa City. Charlie McConnell taught me what even a really bad roofer simply would not do. The usual caveats apply. They taught me a lot and did their best to correct my errors. Those that remain are mine alone.

Brooke Warner, my writing coach and publisher of She Writes Press, helped me walk that line between demonstrating the hypomanic brain and leaving the reader in the dust. Katherine Sharpe tried to correct my grammar and did otherwise fix the manuscript.

My first readers: Mary Vermillion (a real author!) gave me my first encouragement to keep going. John McManamy, Jessica Gimeno, and Joanne Shortell brought my story out of its still-trying-to-sound-sane shell. My readers at ProzacMonologues.com

202 **PROZAC MONOLOGUES**

convinced me I had to keep writing. My friends with depression told me I absolutely had to publish this book.

My book buddies did many and sundry favors that helped me get the job done. Thanks to Kit, Betsy, and Ruth.

And then there's Helen. Always Helen. My words fail.

Thank you.

ABOUT THE AUTHOR

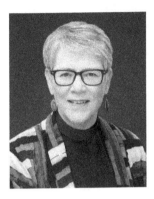

Willa Goodfellow's early work with troubled teens as an Episcopal priest shaped an edgy perspective and preaching style. A bachelor's degree from Reed College and a master's from Yale gave her the intellectual chops to read and comprehend scientific research about mental illness—and her life mileage taught her to recognize and call out the bull.

So she set out to turn her own misbegotten sojourn in the land of antidepressants into a writing career. Her journalism has attracted the attention of leading psychiatrists who worked on the DSM-5. She is certified in Mental Health First Aid, graduated from NAMI's Peer-to-Peer, and has presented on mental health recovery at NAMI events and Carver College of Medicine at the University of Iowa.

Today she hikes, travels, plans seven-course dinner menus, works on her next writing project, *Bar Tales of Costa Rica*, and stirs up trouble. She lives with her wife, Helen, in Central Oregon and still misses her dog Mazie.

Author photo © Vakker Portraits

SELECTED TITLES FROM SHE WRITES PRESS

She Writes Press is an independent publishing company founded to serve women writers everywhere. Visit us at www.shewritespress.com.

A Different Kind of Same: A Memoir by Kelley Clink. $16.95, 978-1-63152-999-3. Several years before Kelley Clink's brother hanged himself, she attempted suicide by overdose. In the aftermath of his death, she traces the evolution of both their illnesses, and wonders: If he couldn't make it, what hope is there for her?

Searching for Normal: The Story of a Girl Gone Too Soon by Karen Meadows. $16.95, 978-1-63152-137-9. Karen Meadows intertwines her own story with excerpts from her daughter Sadie's journals to describes their roller coaster ride through Sadie's depression and a maze of inadequate mental health treatment and services—one that ended with Sadie's suicide at age eighteen.

Off the Rails: One Family's Journey Through Teen Addiction by Susan Burrowes. $16.95, 978-1-63152-467-7. An inspiring story of family love, determination, and the last-resort intervention that helped one troubled young woman find sobriety after a terrifying and harrowing journey.

But My Brain Had Other Ideas: A Memoir of Recovery from Brain Injury by Deb Brandon. $16.95, 978-1631522468. When Deb Brandon discovered that cavernous angiomas—tangles of malformed blood vessels in her brain—were what was behind her the terrifying symptoms she'd been experiencing, she underwent one brain surgery. And then another. And then another. And that was just the beginning.

Learning to Eat Along the Way by Margaret Bendet. $16.95, 978-1-63152-997-9. After interviewing an Indian holy man, newspaper reporter Margaret Bendet follows him in pursuit of enlightenment and ends up facing demons that were inside her all along.

Mothering Through the Darkness: Women Open Up About the Postpartum Experience edited by Stephanie Sprenger and Jessica Smock. $16.95, 978-1-63152-804-0. A collection of thirty powerful essays aimed at spreading awareness and dispelling myths about postpartum depression and perinatal mood disorders.